"In *Practicing Psychotherapy*, Dr. Chamberlain provides a 'true north' for students of psychotherapy and early career professionals, as well as encouragement and a challenge to seasoned professionals. The text offers a compelling argument, illustrated with vivid and moving anecdotes, that our best work depends on continuous development of a special kind of compassion, muscular enough to dismantle outdated concepts ('we' treat 'them') and tender enough to continually nurture our own and others' flawed, brilliant, messy, and creative humanity."

Jonathan Richard, Psy. D., is a Clinical Psychologist in Denver, CO

"Essential book for ANYONE who wants to be—or is—a counselor or therapist! Contemporary mental health training often emphasizes evidenced-based methods matched nicely to diagnoses. It often looks so easy. But this highly structured approach often leaves counselors and therapists unprepared for life 'out there' where there are no manuals or roadmaps. The results can be devastating emotional burnout or much worse. This book may be just the needed antidote. Dr. Chamberlain shows us glimpses of life as a *real* therapist, working with volatile, occasionally joyful, difficult, sometimes ungrateful, and all-too-human clients. Read this book to view the mind and heart of a master clinician as she recounts her journey across the lifespan, with skills that treatment manuals can never teach. Read it again to absorb the clinical wisdom on each page. But most of all, if you believe therapy is your calling, you need to spend time with this book and reflect carefully whether this path is really yours. This lifetime journey is magnificent, but it is not for the faint-of-heart."

Bill McCown, Ph.D., Clinical Psychologist, coordinator, Department of Psychology and associate dean for Research, University of Louisiana at Monroe

"Exceptional book giving insight to the experiences of a psychotherapist! Dr. Chamberlain provides a glimpse into the world of a professional therapist. Clients seek counseling due to various stressors, and this book can help new psychotherapists learn how to be open-minded. Schools of psychotherapy cannot pre-pare students for the various challenges clients may display. Dr. Chamberlain's book is an excellent read for new clinicians in the field of psychotherapy."

Eddie Williams, Ed.D., LMHC, NCC, MCAP, HS-BCP,
program director/assistant professor, Human Services,
Pasco-Hernando State College

PRACTICING PSYCHOTHERAPY

In this book of lessons learned from working as a psychotherapist for over 40 years, Dr. Chamberlain shares her varied expertise and experiences, bestowing the wisdom she has gleaned throughout her career from patients, students, teachers, and colleagues.

The text examines three core themes: How helping clients is often intertwined with the therapist's own life journey; the experience of building intimate relationships with vulnerable populations; and the process of accepting loss, letting go, and moving forward, both for the client and the therapist. Prioritizing personal narratives, case examples, professional research, and discussions with experienced clinicians, this book marks the significant impact psychotherapy has on not just patients and clients but also the mental health professional.

Offering enlightenment for readers ranging from longstanding psychotherapists to former patients, this unique book provides a particularly valuable resource for beginning therapists and therapists-in-training who seek a greater understanding of what it means to be a successful and effective therapist.

Linda L. Chamberlain, Psy.D., is a Licensed Psychologist in private practice and professor of Human Services at Pasco-Hernando State College in New Port Richey, Florida.

PRACTICING PSYCHOTHERAPY

Lessons on Helping Patients and Growing as a Professional

Linda L. Chamberlain

Routledge
Taylor & Francis Group

NEW YORK AND LONDON

First published 2021
by Routledge
52 Vanderbilt Avenue, New York, NY 10017

and by Routledge
2 Park Square, Milton Park, Abingdon, Oxon, OX14 4RN

Routledge is an imprint of the Taylor & Francis Group, an informa business

Library of Congress Cataloging-in-Publication Data

Names: Chamberlain, Linda L., author.
Title: Practicing psychotherapy : lessons on helping patients and growing as a professional/Linda L. Chamberlain.
Description: New York, NY : Routledge, 2021. | Includes bibliographical references and index.
Identifiers: LCCN 2020026331 (print) | LCCN 2020026332 (ebook) | ISBN 9780367373702 (paperback) | ISBN 9780367373672 (hardback) | ISBN 9780429355493 (ebook)
Subjects: LCSH: Psychotherapy. | Psychotherapists--Vocational guidance. | Psychotherapist and patient.
Classification: LCC RC480 .C45 2021 (print) | LCC RC480 (ebook) | DDC 616.89/14--dc23
LC record available at https://lccn.loc.gov/2020026331
LC ebook record available at https://lccn.loc.gov/2020026332

ISBN: 978-0-367-37367-2 (hbk)
ISBN: 978-0-367-37370-2 (pbk)
ISBN: 978-0-429-35549-3 (ebk)

Typeset in Joanna
by KnowledgeWorks Global Ltd.

CONTENTS

PART III
How to Let Go   **105**

PREFACE

In many ways, this is a book that I've been working on for almost 50 years. I started studying Buddhism and psychology at about that same time in my late teens and both have been life-long pursuits. My interest in psychotherapy and Buddhist practice have blended and each has influenced the other. This book is an opportunity for me to weave together the threads of Buddhist thought, my experiences with patients, students and colleagues, and my journey through my career as a psychotherapist.

As a psychotherapist, I've found that Buddhist teachings about how we live, how we love and how we let go are a useful rubric for understanding the life problems that we all face. I also use it to better understand the dilemmas that patients bring to our work together. I've organized this book according to those challenges and how they emerge in the therapy relationship. My encounters in therapy with thousands of people during my career has been an unparalleled opportunity to better appreciate the unique way that each of us use in our life to meet the goals of loving, living, and letting go.

As a writer, quieting myself and struggling with the discipline to sit in contemplation as I write has always been a challenge. I approach writing with a mix of excitement and dread. I'll do anything, even vacuum the cats, before I finally settle myself. Those mornings that begin a day devoted to putting thoughts into words on paper are usually fueled by at least two cups of tea, a game of Sudoku, and checking messages from the previous day. Like many authors, I have a love/hate relationship with writing: I adore it when I'm in the midst of it and resent the time I must devote to it when I could be gardening, reading, kayaking, or spending time with friends. This book, however, is a labor of love and has been a return to the joy that writing brings me. For that, I am so grateful.

It is my hope that this will be a guidebook to those coming into the profession and that more experienced professionals will see some reflection of their experiences in the big chair. I use the "big chair" throughout this book as the symbol for life as a psychotherapist. It's a ubiquitous presence in our lives. The one thing that most psychotherapists don't skimp on is buying a really comfortable, big chair. We spend a lot of time there. Sometimes I wish that my office was in a place that was conducive to walking outdoors as I meet with patients so I could get a bit more exercise during days at the practice. For now, however, it's how most of us work: We sit in the big chair while our patients occupy the couch or other chairs in our office, and we talk.

After all this time, I'm still amazed at the willingness of people who don't know me to come into my office, share things they may never have told anyone else, trust me to keep their confidence, and then pay me. I know what I offer has value and I'm happy I get to make a living doing this, but it still feels odd at times. Over more than a century, the profession of "psychotherapist" has become integrated into our culture and, for the most part, is a respected part of our health care system. People who are uninformed about the nature of psychotherapy often construe it as either getting advice about what to do or having someone read their minds: Two things that, fortunately, I am very poor at doing. What I have become better at, however, is active, compassionate listening. It's the skill that I work hardest to improve because the power of truly listening to someone else can have such a profoundly healing effect.

Throughout the book, I'll share experiences that I found challenging or illuminating. My caveat to the reader is that this is only my journey. If something you read resonates with you, I'm delighted. If something you read has no connection to you, I'm delighted. Please compare what I share with your lived experience, whether you are a student, therapist in training, experienced professional, patient or just curious about psychotherapy.

Take what you need and leave the rest. How I practice is unique to my beliefs, values, experiences, and training. When I read accounts from other authors about life as a psychotherapist, I find that there are entire pages I highlight and occasional chapters that I skim through. In Buddhist teachings, we are warned to not accept any belief or theory that isn't supported by evidence, either from scientific inquiry, application of logic, or our lived experience. I encourage you to approach this book with that in mind.

I'm so grateful to have had so many interesting, life changing experiences throughout my career. I began in the mid-1970s working in a state hospital in Austin, Texas with severely and chronically mentally ill patients. After two years, I moved to San Angelo, Texas, where I worked with a day treatment program and supervised a crisis intervention hot line at a community mental health center. In the early 1980s, I moved to Dallas, Texas and later to Denver, Colorado with a private, inpatient facility for treatment of addiction. By the mid-1980s, I was director of outpatient drug treatment services with a community based, non-profit and began pursuing my Doctorate in Professional Psychology at the University of Denver. After graduating, I worked for two years with a private group practice in Las Vegas, Nevada that focused on treatment of gambling disorders. I returned to Denver in 1991 and was employed in a managed mental health care group practice for two years, then joined a private group practice, the Colorado Family Center, which focused on high conflict child custody cases. In 2004, I moved to Tampa, Florida and was director of the Center for Addiction and Substance Abuse at the University of South Florida student counseling center for 3 years. I have also managed my own private practice both in Denver, Colorado and currently in New Port Richey, Florida. Along with my clinical practice career, I've been on faculty at the University of Nevada, Las Vegas; Regis University and the University of Denver in Denver, Colorado; the University of South Florida in Tampa, Florida; and I am currently a Professor of Human Services at Pasco-Hernando State College in New Port Richey, Florida.

You might notice that I am by nature a seeker of new experiences. I've had the opportunity to work in both the public and private sectors of our profession with a wide array of different populations and issues. Learning something new is what gets me high. I can't think of a boring day since I began this career in the 1970s. I have also had the opportunity to collaborate with others on books and conference presentations with a focus on family therapy, addiction treatment, problem gambling, and applications of chaos, and complexity theory to the practice of psychotherapy. This is my first solo book and I miss the shared experience of writing with others. I plan to return to shared authorship with the next book focused on how being a psychotherapist changes us. I've had such amazing experiences along the way and learned so much. I hope to share some of that with you.

Working with patients is constantly exciting and challenging. At this time, in the midst of the COVID-19 pandemic, I'm learning to adjust to "virtual" psychotherapy sessions on the phone and through Zoom and other video access programs. I'm always learning something through my clinical practice. The more I've attempted to be of help to patients, the more aware I am of how much I have been helped. It's something I didn't expect when I started this career: That I would be changed by the work. Each session challenges me to think about how we, as human beings, face our fears and learn to move our lives in a positive direction. Since I'm a human being too, I get to discover along with my patients ways to change or to accept the challenges that we all face. I hope this book does justice to some of the lives and stories that patients have shared with me. In the book, I've described encounters with some of my patients, all of which have been amended by combining several patient's stories or changing identifying information. If, by chance, a former patient is reading this book and recognizes something, I hope that my respect and appreciation for our work together is clear. I share those stories to honor the work that we did together and as thanks for what I learned.

Most importantly, I hope that you enjoy this book. I've certainly enjoyed living the life that allowed me to write it. Even though I'm still active in teaching and practicing psychotherapy, at 68 years old, I'm feeling more devoted to being of help to those who are beginning their careers. I get such pleasure out of consulting with colleagues and training students who are finding their way into this profession. I'm always happy to hear from former students or interns who have also found this career to be so meaningful. It's good to know that when I finally decide to vacate the big chair and spend more time in my garden and traveling to visit friends that there are such dedicated, talented people to take over.

ACKNOWLEDGMENTS

I'm deeply grateful to the patients who have entrusted me with their care over the decades. So many of the people I've met while in the big chair have had an indelible impact on me. I can only hope that our encounter was as helpful to you as it was to me. I could not have better teachers of patience, compassion, courage, determination, acceptance, and endurance. Thank you.

My students continue to be a source of deep joy. Nothing makes me happier than hearing from a student who is now working in the field and is passionately devoted to the people they serve. I look forward every day to our work together in the classroom helping students build a life in this profession. I learn something from my students every day. I hope one day to be reading your books and going to your talks at conferences. I could not have had better teachers of hope, hard work, commitment, resilience, and dedication. Thank you.

I owe my colleagues so much. Dr. Michael Bütz was instrumental in getting me off my couch and back to my desk to start writing again. Next book, we'll work together again, I hope. Dr. William McCown and Dr. Jon Richard, longtime friends and colleagues, helped this book become a reality and offered suggestions and advice that was enormously helpful in guiding me. Talks with my office mates, Erika Remsberg and Paloma SparrowHawk, inspire and encourage me. Thank you.

I appreciate the faculty and administration at Pasco-Hernando State College who approved a sabbatical to support me writing this book. I'm grateful to all the college staff and administrators who gave me the time to focus on this endeavor, especially Dr. Eddie Williams, Dr. Billie Gabbard, Suzanne Ackerman, Sonia Thorn, Dr. Stan Giannet and Dr. Timothy Beard. Thank you.

I am very grateful for other psychotherapists who have written so eloquently about psychotherapy and Buddhist philosophy. Jack Kornfield's book The Wise Heart is one that I never stop reading. As soon as I finish, I begin again. Reading Jeffrey Kottler and Irving Yalom's wise and eloquent books often made me feel that everything that could be written about life as a psychotherapist had already been written. The works uniting Buddhist thought and psychotherapy by Jon Carlson, Lorne Ladner, Marsha Linehan, Steven Hick, and Thomas Bien also served as guides and inspiration in my work on this book. Namaste' and thank you.

My editors at Routledge, Nina Guttapalle, and Grace McDonnell and their staff were a pleasure to work with and offered invaluable advice during the process of writing this book. I am so grateful for your patience, guidance, and assistance. Thank you.

Finally, thanks to my partner and one of the best writers I know, Jeff McBee. It's lovely to share a home with someone who knows his grammar and punctuation and can make a pizza entirely from scratch (I think I smell the sauce cooking right now). I appreciate your proof-reading and editing help and for picking up the chores I didn't get to on days that I just wanted to read and write. Also, for sharing the writing table in the most beautiful spot on earth, your cottage on Lake Skootamatta. Thank you.

PART I
HOW TO LIVE

The chapters in this section focus on the question, "What makes for a good life"? How to live is the first challenge in Buddhist philosophy. We have a human life, now what do we intend to do with it? Everyone shares the struggle to survive, to become a good person, and to find some meaning and fulfillment in their lives. As we work at helping others meet that challenge, we are faced with the same questions: "Who am I? What do I want? What's in my way?" (Gottlieb, 2019). Psychotherapy isn't just something we do, it's something we enter into along with our clients. We're all on the same journey to build a life we can live with all our heart.

This section offers some guidance to students, trainees, and those in the early part of their career as a psychotherapist. After more than four decades in the big chair, I hope that some of the information and observations that I share can assist in establishing a professional identity and building life skills that will help others in this profession. There are both attitudes and practices that are integral parts of maintaining a long and satisfying career. I will share with you what helped me not only stay in this profession but make a living and build a life for which I am deeply grateful.

Psychotherapy requires as much courage, effort, and determination on the part of the therapist as it does for the patient. It's important, I think, to appreciate that this is one of the hardest jobs anyone could choose. "Every working day holds for us a confrontation with the issues we fear most" (Kottler, 2017, p. 44). Doing the work of a therapist will challenge you. I assure you, over time, this job will also change you, hopefully for the better. If you stay in the big chair over a long career, it can teach you how to live a more compassionate, authentic, and generous life.

There are four chapters in this section that focus on different aspects of learning to make a life in the big chair. The chapters are:

- **Chapter 1: There's Only Us:** This chapter will focus on the dilemma of stigma for populations that psychotherapists often serve. Those of us who suffer from addiction and mental illness are not only challenged by the illness, but by public misunderstanding and the experience of rejection and isolation.
- **Chapter 2: Follow the Yellow Brick Road:** The story The Wizard of Oz provides a framework for defining our human condition. The problems that the characters in the story struggle through reflect concerns we all face: How do I learn to think? How do I learn to feel? How do I learn to act? How do I find my place in the world? I find this story a useful framework for understanding the nature of the problems that patients present.
- **Chapter 3: The Pursuit of Happiness:** This chapter addresses the question of what constitutes happiness? We all desire happiness. The question really is not how we find happiness, but how we create it in our lives. As therapists, we need a deep appreciation of what makes for a happy life if we are to assist others in having a more realistic and successful approach to that pursuit. For those in this profession, learning to maintain a positive mind when faced with so many who are suffering is a requirement for a life in the big chair.
- **Chapter 4: No Matter Where You Go, There You Are:** Over time, guiding others toward better, more positive lives also challenges therapists to evaluate who we are and how we feel about ourselves and our relationships. The importance of being "genuine" with others in therapy requires self-examination and confronting those aspects of who we are that create dilemmas. Since psychotherapy is a shared experience between patient and therapist, it is vital to engage in an ongoing examination of what we bring to that encounter.

Ladner (2004) notes that in Buddhist philosophy, having a "good, happy life is determined not by anything external but rather by the quality of our minds and hearts in each moment of life." (p. 8). I hope that these chapters offer some worthwhile ideas about cultivating a curious, calm, and compassionate mind as the foundation for being of help to others.

1

THERE'S ONLY US

There's Only Us

Several years ago, I attended a conference for human services students and practitioners. About 40 of us were seated in a small meeting room listening to a presentation. I don't remember the specific topic, but the speaker was talking about people with mental illnesses, like depression and anxiety, and how, as therapists, we could best help them. It was the type of talk that is ubiquitous at these conferences. I had facilitated numerous trainings and classes that were much the same: "Here's how *we* help *them*." Then something unusual happened. A young man seated behind me in the audience raised his hand about halfway through the talk and asked a very simple question: "Why are we talking about 'them' when it's really just 'us'?"

Both the speaker and many of us in the audience were initially perplexed by what he was asking. When the speaker asked if he could explain what he meant by the question, the young man shared that he was a student in training to be a social worker and was experiencing a significant bout with depression for the first time in his life. As he was listening to the speaker, he kept hearing how "we," the helpers, were separate from "them," those with mental illness. Because it was his first time attending a conference like this and he was newly diagnosed with depression, he was acutely aware of how the "us" and "them" dichotomy was affecting him. I remember clearly his statement that "It makes me question whether I belong here." What happens in our field when we pose as "the well" and our patients as "the sick?"

Fortunately, the speaker was wise enough to change the focus of her talk to the concern the young man raised. The rest of the time was spent in dialogue among the participants about his question. I recall that many in the audience also shared their struggles with some type of emotional challenge, mental illness, grief, addiction, heartbreak, or fear. It was both an outpouring of support for the young man and a cathartic experience for many of us. Although many of the older professionals in the audience had known each other for years, we had rarely shared our own experiences and struggles. As the discussion progressed, it became clear that there were only "us" in the room, no "them."

After that meeting, there was a greater feeling of connection and compassion during the rest of the conference. Talks over dinner became more personal and emotionally intimate; deeper friendships were formed. I remember a sense of relief at being able to step out of my professional persona and get better acquainted with colleagues. There was such freedom in putting aside my role as therapist and being more "me." Many of our students who attended the conference expressed their gratitude at hearing their mentors and professors openly sharing some of their personal struggles. It helped to relieve them of the sense that they couldn't be in the profession if they had a history of addiction or mental health problems.

I often think of that young man with deep gratitude for his courage in speaking up that afternoon. His comment profoundly changed my awareness and challenged me to be more authentic about my experiences. I am more acutely aware of my language when I am teaching or training students or speaking as a professional in public. Stigma profoundly complicates what is already a complex challenge for those of us with mental illness. That's how I talk about it now: Those of us. Yalom (2002) writes, "I prefer to think of my patients and myself as *fellow travelers*, a term that abolishes distinctions between 'them' ('the afflicted') and 'us' (the healers)" (p. 8). One of the effects of the young man's statement was that it encouraged me to be more open about my experiences. I now weave his lesson, that there is only "us," into my classes and presentations at conferences. I often felt as though my professors, mentors, and colleagues in the field were somehow able to transcend the human condition. As I became the therapist, teacher, and trainer, I also adopted that mask. Even with friends, I rarely shared my own challenges with anxiety and depression. I perpetuated the stigma around mental illness by creating the impression that I had never been personally affected. "Therapists, of course, deal with the daily challenges of living just like everyone else" (Gottlieb, 2019). That statement is true for all of us in the big chair.

My other teacher on the subject of "us" was renowned psychotherapist Carl Rogers. His book On Becoming a Person (Rogers, 1961) had significantly influenced my philosophy of human nature when I was working on my master's degree in counseling psychology in the late 1970s. I was fortunate to hear him speak at the first "Evolution of Psychotherapy" conferences in 1985 in Phoenix, Arizona. He was talking about his life as a researcher, teacher, and therapist. He had shared several of the seminal experiences that had shaped his work, many of which I was familiar with from his writings. He also shared a recent experience that became another awakening for me regarding the "us" and "them" dilemma. Not long before the conference, Dr. Rogers' wife had died. He talked about the enormous impact of the loss and the profound grief he experienced. He was still an active professional and continued to work following her death. His grief was sometimes overwhelming. What I was most struck by was his description of how isolated he felt. He was the teacher, master therapist, and mentor; it would be inappropriate to bring his own experience to the forefront. He described, however, that one day a student noticed his sadness and simply asked him "Can I help?" Dr. Rogers shared his deep gratitude that someone had been willing to ask him if he was alright and to offer him compassion and an opportunity to talk about his grief. He was invited to just be a human being who was in a painful time and to share that with another person.

I was grateful for his willingness to share that experience with the hundreds of us who attended his talk. It became clear to me that regardless of the level to which we rise professionally, there's only us: Human beings who endure suffering. I had often debated whether to share some of my experiences with depression and anxiety with my students and had always chosen not to. I instead maintained the aura of mastery and "professional-ism." Dr. Rogers' description of how isolating and difficult it was to contain his grief and the appreciation he had for the student who showed him com-passion encouraged me to step out of the role of teacher and be a human being. Now, when I facilitate classes on "Abnormal Psychology" (one of my least favorite course titles) or "Issues in Mental Health," I tell my students about my history of panic attacks and periods of depression. We talk about "us." We discuss the dilemma of stigma around mental illness and how we can have a positive impact when we become more open about our own experiences.

Overcoming Stigma

Who hasn't been impacted by either their own or a loved one's struggles with mental illness? Stigma silences many of us. During classroom discus-sions, some of my students openly share their challenges with addiction, mental illness, or trauma. I am always grateful for their willingness to openly confront the stigma. I appreciate how brave they are in taking a risk to share their stories. I usually start that discussion by asking who in the class knows someone who has a mental illness or addiction? Most students raise their hands. For those who don't, I approach them and shake their hand and introduce myself; "I'm Linda Chamberlain and I have a history of panic disorder and dysthymia. I'm glad to meet you." That way, I can be sure that everyone knows someone who has experienced a mental disorder.

For many years, my concern was whether I would be considered an effective, competent mental health professional and teacher if I admitted that I have experienced mental illness. When I began to share more about my history of panic attacks and depression, I was grateful for the under-standing and support that students extended to me. Sharing my experience gave them a chance to ask questions and for us to have a dialogue about mental illness on a more personal level. The silence was broken. Now, it isn't "us" and "them," there is only us. We know that other health profes-sionals become ill; doctors get the flu and dentists have cavities. Many of us who work with mental illness and addiction have suffered from those disorders, but it's rare that we disclose our stories. It's the stigma around mental health and addiction that keeps us silent for so long. I think our willingness as mental health professionals to share some of our personal experiences can help better shape our students and trainees by encouraging them to be more open and proactive if they experience a mental illness. It certainly reminds us that we are a part of, not apart from, the human condition.

One way that we began to address stigma on our campus at Pasco-Hernando State College (PHSC) involved working with several of my students to form a chapter of NAMI (National Alliance on Mental Illness) on Campus to make our small college a more welcoming and supportive environment for those of us who have experienced a psychological challenge. Although we partner with a local community mental health center, our college doesn't have a counseling service on campus. One of the problems that is frequently raised by staff and faculty is the question of how to deal with a student who was having a mental health crisis. Since I'm a clinical psychologist, it was not unusual for coworkers to consult with me about someone in their classes who was clearly experiencing emotional or behavioral difficulties. Research suggests that anxiety disorders and depression are much more prevalent in college populations (Corey et.al, 2012). It's rare to have a class of 20 students and not have at least a few of them approach me at some point in the semester to share their struggles with a mental health problem.

I also invite speakers who are willing to share their stories about addiction or mental illness. Former students, members of our staff and faculty, and representatives from NAMI have been generous with their time in talking with my classes. I also search for videos and films that feature people living with mental disorders or recovering from addiction. Two of the films that I recommend are "A Beautiful Mind" and "The Soloist." Both provide excellent depictions of someone with a serious mental illness and how they are helped by others who care about their welfare. They also address how stigma and fear are impediments in coping effectively with a mental disorder. I'm a fan of Ted Talks and some that I share with students are Elyn Saks (June, 2012), "A tale of mental illness – from the inside," Sangu Delle (February, 2017), "There's no shame in taking care of your mental health," and Johann Hari (June, 2015), "Everything you think you know about addiction is wrong." Each of these Ted Talks presenters helps to raise awareness and confront stigma. I'm so grateful for the wealth of compelling and compassionate voices that are now being raised to help establish an environment of understanding and support. If we learn to see beyond the fear, pain, and confusion, we inevitably find a being like us who desires to give and receive compassion and understanding. Stigma is born of and nourished by ignorance and fear, familiarity and information about mental illness and addiction helps us reduce the harm stigma causes.

The first of the Four Noble Truths in Buddhist philosophy is that everyone suffers (Claxton, 1999). For addiction and mental illness, stigma and isolation turn pain into suffering. We can help to mitigate that. Pain is unavoidable in life, but suffering can be managed and reduced by connection to others. It is painful when someone we love leaves us, but it creates suffering when we believe that loss means we are un-lovable or doomed to be lonely forever. Suffering is how we describe to ourselves the meaning of pain in a way that diminishes us. Pain wounds us, but suffering prevents the wound from healing. We can't create a life free of painful experiences, but we can learn to reduce the degree of our suffering when we share that pain in conversation with others. Helping people reduce the suffering that we create as a response to pain is the very foundation of the practice of psychotherapy.

NOTES FROM THE BIG CHAIR

Over the course of four decades in this profession, it has become clear to me that our painful, challenging experiences are the foundation for developing compassion. Certainly, not everyone finds the path through crisis and confusion that leads to a greater capacity for caring. Pain, however, can be a terrific teacher. It shatters illusions and opens doors to connect with others who have suffered. Difficult experiences are raw materials that build meaningful lives and relationships. It's the pain we endure that brings us to see a therapist and to seek a better understanding of what's happening in our lives. Often, those hurtful experiences are the impetus for people to pursue a career as a therapist: That desire to pass on to others the help that they received or to assure that others get the help that wasn't there for them. We address not only our individual suffering but become committed to reducing the suffering of others.

I'm always aware of the importance of being present for my patients and not diverting their attention to my experiences. It's a cardinal rule, and rightly so, that the person in the big chair doesn't take center stage. Therapy is not about the therapist; the patient's needs are always the focus. There are those moments, however, when we can say "I know how it feels to be scared...to be rejected...to be lonely...to feel hopeless...to feel lost." Empathy is compassion in action. I know from my experience on the couch when I've sought help just how healing it can be to have someone who is willing to be with me in my confusion and hurt. Being in the presence of a compassionate person – someone who can bear witness – is a powerful experience. To feel that we are not alone, that someone cares about our well-being, is how suffering is mitigated. That's the work we've chosen to do as therapists.

I appreciate all the techniques and innovative approaches that we have developed over the years to help people. I have seen quite a few therapy orientations and different methodologies or techniques come and go (anyone today practicing Primal Scream Therapy?). I've certainly tried many different strategies to be of help to my patients, from Eye Movement Desensitization and Reprocessing (EMDR) (Shapiro, 2018) to mindfulness training. My experience, however, is that there is nothing more effective than focusing on our shared human condition. "Each time we meet another human being and honor their dignity, we help those around us" (Kornfield, 2008, p. 17). The first lesson in becoming an effective therapist is to learn to be respectful and to appreciate that everyone you will encounter in your career is a suffering human being, just as you are.

It's my hope that when we sit in the big chair, we don't forget our connection to the joys and sorrows of our own experience. Without that awareness and appreciation of our happiness and suffering, how do we connect in a meaningful way to those experiences in others? We are tasked with helping not only individuals but our larger world to become a better place for all of us, regardless of our unique history. I believe that an important goal of psychotherapy is to help us cope with pain in a manner that doesn't increase our suffering. Through acknowledging our own challenging experiences and how we have learned to cope, we share hope and reduce stigma.

Lessons from the Big Chair: Chapter 1

- Relate to people, not diagnoses.
- Use inclusive language when talking about mental health and addiction. Avoid the "us" and "them" dichotomy.
- Honor the dignity of all you meet; each person you encounter has something to teach you.
- Keep yourself human and humble. If you haven't experienced a dilemma that therapy could help with, you will.

Case Study: Me

I share with my students how I was impacted by panic attacks when I was just starting in private practice after completing my doctorate degree at the University of Denver in 1989. I was in my mid-thirties, living in Las Vegas, Nevada with my husband of several years and working in a group practice. In the first year that I lived in Las Vegas, I was confronted with several significant challenges. My husband stated that he "just needed space" and we separated at his request just a few months after I arrived. I tried to be supportive of my husband's need for "space" even though we had been separated for almost 6 months prior to my coming to join him in Las Vegas after he took a job there while I was completing my doctoral internship year in Denver. For reasons I didn't understand, I was alone in a large house in a city where I didn't know anyone. I was hurt and confused, but he assured me he just needed to sort some things out in his life and didn't want to end the marriage.

Work became my refuge. I didn't have a social life or people to spend time with outside of my colleagues at the office. I was happy to take on additional cases. It was a busy practice, so taking on 8 to 10 clients a day, 5 days a week wasn't hard to do. I was learning how to work with problem gambling which, given my background in addiction treatment, was intriguing and challenging. I was grateful to finally be making a good living in a job for which I had spent years training. That part of my life was stimulating and deeply satisfying. I was doing well professionally; my career aspirations were becoming reality. Every night, however, I went home to a big empty house. There was no one to share my day with and I felt profoundly alone for the first time.

In late 1990, my father died very suddenly and unexpectedly of a heart attack. I was graced with a father who was devoted to our family. He was a kind, hard-working, loving man who I adored. I spent time with him in the garage building bookcases and sailboats; fashioning skateboards from a piece of plywood and my old roller skates. He taught me to run a table saw and read wood-working plans before I could boil an egg or do a load of laundry. My favorite story about him is how he responded to my confusion when I had to write a report in 4th grade about what I wanted to be when I grew up. I had gone to the library (as I loved to do) and found two books (and only two) about women who had a career: One about Amelia Earhart and the other about Madame Marie Curie. After reading them, I told my dad I didn't really know which one I wanted to be, an aviator or a scientist. My father had flown in World War II and offered to loan me his aviator's cap if I wanted to write about being a pilot, which is what I did. When I got home after school on the day that I gave the report, however, I went into my room and there was a microscope on my desk. I was thrilled! When my father came home from work and I went to thank him, he grinned and said, "I couldn't afford to get you an airplane, but I could get you a microscope." So began my love of science. When he died, I lost my most treasured source of love and support.

I returned to Texas for the funeral. My mother, younger brother, and grandmother (my father's mother) who lived with us were all devastated. It was the first time someone I loved had died. After a week with family, I went back to work in Las Vegas. In February 1991, I was meeting late one evening with a new client. I was the last one in the office that night. Suddenly, I felt like I had been slammed in the chest with a sledgehammer. I couldn't breathe and was in terrible pain. As I gasped for air and curled up on the floor of the office, I was aware how horrified the client was about what was happening to me. She was panicked by my behavior, but able to call 911 at my request. She stayed until the ambulance arrived. Not surprisingly, that was the last time I saw her despite trying a few days later to reach her to reschedule.

Tests at the hospital confirmed that my heart was fine. What I imagined a heart attack would feel like was instead a panic attack. It was the first of several more that I would experience in the coming months. I stopped staying late at the office as the second attack also occurred there just a few days later after seeing my last client for the night. Until then, I had only sat in the big chair in a therapy office, but it was clear that I now needed some time on the couch. One of my colleagues in the practice referred me to a wonderful therapist who was enormously helpful in guiding me to an understanding of what was happening and what the panic attacks might be trying to tell me. Being a patient was the best training I ever had in how to be a good therapist. I'm grateful for becoming an "us," even though it took me years to openly acknowledge my experience.

2

FOLLOW THE YELLOW BRICK ROAD

Finding the Yellow Brick Road

In one of my first psychology courses as an undergraduate at the University of Texas in 1972, I asked a professor to recommend a book to help me understand psychotherapy. I had never been to consult with a therapist and didn't have a clear sense of what took place between a therapist and client. It was like a black box; someone went in, something happened, and they emerged a different person in some way. So, what happened? How did therapy work? What brought someone to see a therapist and what did the therapist do? In the early 1970s, there were very few popular depictions of psychotherapy in movies or on television. The "Bob Newhart Show" in which Bob Newhart played a psychotherapist was my template for what therapists did. I had only one friend who had seen a therapist and I was always reluctant to ask her about what she experienced. For me, therapy was a mystery and therapists were even more mysterious.

I asked the professor, "If I want to understand what a therapist does, what should I read?" The professor looked thoughtful, grinned and said read

The Wonderful Wizard of Oz. As a child, I loved the annual screening of the Judy Garland movie musical version, The Wizard of Oz. I knew the story, but the professor instructed me to read the original work. He encouraged me to be curious about the questions of why people sought out therapy and what a therapist does to help clients. I found a copy of Frank Baum's (1900) original book. As I read the story, I kept my professor's instructions in mind. I loved the story and I reread that book every few years. In my introductory courses on therapeutic skills, I still recommend that students read the original story. For me, the yellow brick road provides a map of both what brings people to therapy and what heals them. It also provides an interesting perspective on my original question of what therapists do to be of help to others.

The Wonderful Wizard of Oz

In the original text, Baum describes writing the story as a "…modernized fairy tale, in which the wonderment and joy are retained, and the heart-aches and nightmares are left out" (1900, p. v). If that was his aspiration, he certainly fell short of the goal. The story is filled with terror and loss. In fact, the entire story is Dorothy's nightmare. Each of the characters in her dream goes with her to seek the Wizard because of their own heartache. The characters who are journeying on the yellow brick road are seeking help to gain a missing part of themselves. The road to Oz leads Dorothy and her companions, the Scarecrow, the Tin Man, and the Lion, on a journey of healing and enlightenment. They are all seeking the help of the Wizard because Dorothy was told that he could be of help in fulfilling her desire to go home again. It's a journey of faith that there is someone they can meet who will show them how to be whole and happy by granting their requests for a home, a brain, a heart, and courage. Although I trust most readers are familiar with the story, we'll follow the yellow brick road as a map that guides us through the questions: Why do people come to therapy? How do people heal? What is a therapist's role?

The tale begins with Dorothy, a young orphaned girl, who is living with her Aunt Em and Uncle Harry on the bleak, gray, empty plains of Kansas in a tiny one-room house. Her sole companion is her dog, Toto, who provides the only happiness she knows. We don't know why Dorothy was orphaned or how long she's lived with the joyless Aunt Em and grim, hardworking Uncle Harry. Her existence is as bleak and gray as the landscape. A cyclone suddenly blows in from the north and Dorothy is unable to get to the safety of the cellar because she can't catch Toto. Consequently, Dorothy and Toto are caught inside the spinning house that is being carried along by the storm.

> "At first, she had wondered if she would be dashed to pieces when the house fell again: But as the hours passed and nothing terrible happened, she stopped worrying and resolved to wait calmly and see what the future would bring" (Baum, 1900, p. 4).

A terrible event has ripped Dorothy away from everything that is familiar to her. She faces the crisis with fear and, finally, resignation. Anyone whose life has been thrown into turmoil by a catastrophic event can understand her reaction. It's often an overwhelming experience that brings people to therapy, whether it's the loss of safety and security, the end of a relationship, an illness or injury, or traumatic experiences. Dorothy is in crisis and fears that her world will never be the same again. As her fears begin to calm, she falls asleep.

Dorothy awakens when the house lands in Oz, a place populated by very unusual people, the Munchkins. They celebrate her as a liberator because her house lands on and kills an evil witch who has enslaved them for many years. Although they are kind to her and invite her to live in their community, Dorothy wants nothing more than to go home, to be back where she belongs. They tell her about the Wizard of Oz who might be able to help her but warn that it is a "long journey, through a country that is sometimes pleasant and sometimes dark and terrible" (Baum, 1900, p. 10). They also instruct her that "When you get to Oz, do not be afraid of him, but tell your story and ask him to help you" (p. 11). Just "follow the yellow brick road" is good advice to anyone seeking therapy: It will sometimes be a pleasant experience but also dark and difficult. Don't let your fear stop you from seeking what you desire and telling your story.

Dorothy sets off with Toto to find the Wizard. She knows that if she wants to get home, she must pass through rough and dangerous places before she can feel safe and secure, before she feels at home again. As she's walking, she meets a Scarecrow and tells him about the Wizard. The Scarecrow explains he has only straw instead of brains in his head and that his dearest desire is to be able to have a brain. "I do not want people to call me a fool, and if my head stays stuffed with straw instead of with brains, as yours is, how am I ever to know anything?" (p. 17). He sets off with Dorothy in the hope that the Wizard can give him a brain so that he can solve problems, make plans, and better understand his world. The Scarecrow repeatedly falls into holes in the yellow brick road because he can't think clearly enough to avoid repeating the same mistakes. He wants to understand his life more fully. He tells Dorothy that it is "worth a lot of bother to be able to think properly" (p. 24). The Scarecrow wants to think.

As they follow the road, they come upon a Tin Man in the woods who has been immobilized by rust for more than a year. He sadly tells them that "… no one has ever heard me before or come to help me" (p. 25). He shares his story. He was a human who once had brains and a heart and "…having tried them both, I should much rather have a heart" (p. 28). He was in love with a young woman whom he wished to marry but was cursed by the Wicked Witch of the East who enchanted his ax so that when he swung it, he would cut apart his body instead of the trees. A kind tinsmith helped replace his arms, legs, head, and, finally, his body that was split in half, destroying his heart. That was his greatest loss; he could no longer feel love and without that, he could not be happy. He tells them, "…brains do not make one happy, and happiness is the best thing in the world" (p. 30). The Tin Man is hopeful that the Wizard is someone who can help him feel again and give and receive love. His desire is for the Wizard to give him a heart so he can connect to others and experience the happiness that our hearts desire. The Tin Man wants to feel.

Finally, as Dorothy, the Scarecrow, and Tin Man follow the road, they encounter a Lion who threatens Toto. Dorothy confronts the lion by slapping him on the nose and the Lion immediately withdraws. He tells them that he is a coward who is ashamed of his fears, a cowardly Lion. He described his cowardice as a mystery and that "I suppose I was born that way" (p. 33). He feels that his life is "…simply unbearable without a bit of courage" (p. 34) and so decides to go on the journey in the hope that the Wizard can give him bravery in order to do what he needs so he can claim his rightful place in the world as the King of Beasts. He wants to be free of the crippling anxiety that imprisons him. The Lion wants to act without fear.

A minor but important incident happens as they set out together; the Tin Man accidentally steps on a bug and kills it. He begins to weep which rusts his mouth shut. He is overcome with feelings. It is the Scarecrow who understands the problem and seizes the oil can to help the Tin Man. The Scarecrow thinks of the solution to the problem of the Tin Man's heartfelt sorrow at accidentally harming another being.

The Tin Man tells them, "You people with hearts…have something to guide you and need never do wrong, but I don't have a heart, and so I must be very careful. When Oz gives me a heart, of course, I needn't mind so much" (p. 36). Both the Scarecrow and the Tin Man behave in the ways that they wish to: The Scarecrow solves the problem through thinking and the Tin Man cries because he feels so deeply about harming another creature. Later in the story, the Lion takes enormous risks to protect the others. He carries them on his back as he leaps over a ditch and declares "I am terribly afraid of falling…but I suppose there is nothing to do but try it" (p. 39). He acts with courage to help his friends. This pattern of Dorothy's companions behaving in ways they believe they cannot repeats throughout the book. Each demonstrates that they are capable of what they say they aren't.

When the companions finally reach the Emerald City and are ushered individually to meet with the Great Oz, the Wizard appears in a different form to each of them. The Wizard understands that each of his "patients" would need something different from him. To each of them, however, he gave the same assignment. Before he would grant their requests, they had to go on an arduous, perilous journey to free the Land of Oz from the Wicked Witch of the West. Once the journey was complete, he would provide them with the desired brain, heart, courage, and home. And so, after thinking the great Wizard would give them what they wanted, they are sent out without a map to wander through dark woods and fragile landscapes to confront their fears. With each other's help, they vanquish the Wicked Witch. The journey leaves them bruised and exhausted, but proud they were able to do as the Wizard asked. Now, they will finally get what each of them wants.

When they return to Oz after their journey to kill the Witch, rather than finding an all-powerful being who can fix their problems, the Wizard is revealed to be an old man from Omaha who accidentally landed in Oz many years ago. He admits that he can't keep his promises to them, and when Dorothy confronts him and calls him a "bad man" he replies, "Oh no, my dear; I'm a very good man, but I'm a very bad Wizard, I must admit" (p. 107). When the Scarecrow asks, "Can't you give me brains?" he replies, "You don't need them…Experience is the only thing that brings knowledge" (p. 107). To the Tin Man, he says "I think you are wrong to want a heart. It makes most people unhappy" (p. 108). To the Lion, he says

"You have plenty of courage...All you need is confidence in yourself...The true courage is in facing danger when you are afraid..." (p. 108). He does, however, go through a ceremony with the Scarecrow, Tin Man, and Lion in which he gives each of them something symbolic of what they were seeking. He confirms that they now have what they came to get but makes it clear that they accomplished their goals through their own efforts, not his. The items he gives them are like medals they earned through their actions on the journey.

Dorothy is the only one left without getting what she wants: To be home again. Finding our place in the world and creating a life that we can thrive in, our "home," is the most difficult challenge of all. His attempt to take Dorothy back to Kansas fails and Dorothy must set out to see if the good Witch, Glinda, can help her. Once again, she sets off with her companions. After more hardships, Dorothy reaches her destination and finds Glinda, who tells her she always had the power to go home whenever she wanted. Before she goes, however, the Scarecrow, Tin Man, and Lion all recognize how important she has been to them; that without her, they would still be stuck in the dilemmas they had when she first encountered them. "This is all true," said Dorothy, "and I am glad I was of use to these good friends. But now that each of them has had what they most desired, and each one is happy.... I think I should like to go back to Kansas" (p. 144). And she does.

The Scarecrow, Tin Man, and Lion represent what brings people to see a therapist. Our traditional theoretical orientations reflect the dilemmas they embody: Cognitive therapy for the Scarecrow, humanistic therapy for the Tin Man, and behavioral therapy for the Lion. The Scarecrow believes he can't think in effective ways. He lacks the cognitive skills to understand and solve his problems. He can't trust his thoughts to be helpful and result in good outcomes. The Tin Man is lonely and wants to feel love and happiness. He longs to connect to others through his emotions. The Lion can't act because of his fear. He aspires to be courageous enough to do what he wants in the world instead of hiding and avoiding. We have a variety of yellow brick roads to offer our patients; we just need to understand the barriers that keep them from what they are seeking. We can't give patients what they want, but we can help them find their brain, heart, and courage by accompanying them on their journey. Most importantly, along the way, we can point out how they already demonstrate those characteristics they wish to incorporate. It's important to be watchful for the stories or behaviors that contradict the narrative of no brain, no heart, and no courage. When I find them, my goal is to immediately call the patient's attention to those experiences that contradict their self-perceptions. In the process, we help them come home to a life they can live more fully.

Psychotherapists: The Wizard or Dorothy?

Having been a patient, I hoped that I would encounter in my therapist a Wizard who would simply tell me the secret that would solve my problems. Yalom (2002) notes that patients often have "...the happy belief that the therapist knows the way home – a clear, sure path out of pain" (p. 99). Patients project their hopes and fears onto therapists. There is always transference. add Will he be my demanding father? My patient, kind teacher? My loving but ineffectual mother? My abusive partner? Therapists represent something different to each client and part of the work is to understand who we appear to be to those we encounter in therapy. Regardless of our philosophical orientation to psychotherapy, transference exists and impacts the work that we do. We are there to fulfill some desire that the patient brings and there are always expectations about who we are and how we'll treat those who come to us.

I assume that most patients, even those who are familiar with being in therapy, wish that their therapist would fix whatever's broken. Just tell me what to do! I want to be fixed and I've been told you're a great therapist and you can give me what I need. "Those who desire magic, mystery, and authority are loath to look beneath the trappings of the therapist" (Yalom, 2017, p. 99). Like the Wizard, we don't have answers that will instantly unlock a solution. Patients must be willing to go into the dark and frightening places, to explore the damaged, delicate, unacknowledged parts of themselves. We've got to be willing to go through the woods with them and we both must trust that we are able to set out together on a journey that will be uncomfortable, frightening, and sometimes painful. Like our patients, we must take on the challenging task of confronting those aspects of ourselves that are causing pain and creating hurtful patterns in our life. The journey is the solution. It's while we're on the yellow brick road, or lost in the woods, that we discover who we are and gain the experiences that awaken our intelligence, compassion, and courage. It's through our relationships with each other that we create our home. Most importantly, we help each other and, in the process, build better expressions of who we are.

Dorothy is the real wizard. Unlike the Wizard, she embodies Rogers' (1961) observation that "...I have found that it does not help, in the long run, to act as through I were something that I am not" (p. 16). Although clients often are looking for the Wizard if they're fortunate, they find Dorothy in the big chair instead. While they may hope that we will be infinitely patient, all knowing, good natured and calm, and that we'll never be forgetful or ill, it usually doesn't take long to dissuade patients of that fantasy. It is Dorothy who's innate, compassionate concern for the Scarecrow, Tin Man, and Lion encourages them to get on the road to seek what they most need to be whole. When they share what they desire, she invites them to go with her to find what they are seeking. She travels with them as a guide and companion, even as she is on her own journey. She supports their efforts without interference; she consoles them when they are hurt and celebrates when they are victorious. Dorothy makes sure that they care for each other along the way and doesn't let anyone struggle alone. They go where they need to in order to have the experiences that will help them. It's the journey that heals. Dorothy, however, provided the single most important element: Hope. It's the first thing we all need to convince ourselves to follow the yellow brick road wherever it might lead. Dorothy was the companion on the yellow brick road who both helped the others change and, in the process, was herself changed.

NOTES FROM THE BIG CHAIR

Each time I read "*The Wonderful Wizard of Oz*," I find that it offers me something different. I suspect that's because *I'm* different each time I read it. As I grow nearer to the end of my career, I find myself being more sympathetic to the Wizard. After Dorothy declares him a "bad man" for not keeping his promises to them, he abjectly admits that "I'm really a good man, but I'm a very bad Wizard, I must admit." (p. 107). When I first came into this profession, I imagined I could become the

Wizard, the all-knowing, all powerful, wonderful being who would help patients be thoughtful, loving, and brave. I would help them be more at home in the world. I would be clever enough to unlock the fears that trapped patients in their suffering. I would offer elegant solutions to all my patient's concerns.

It took me a long time to understand the power of being kind, patient, hopeful, and committed to the path wherever it would lead my companions and me. I hope that I can continue to develop those qualities and bring them to my encounters with others, whether I'm in my office, a classroom, or sharing a meal with friends. It's been liberating to not be the Wizard and instead be a fellow traveler. There are dark days on the road and days filled with fields of beautiful, intoxicating flowers. I'm not worried about getting to the Emerald City anymore, I prefer to enjoy my companions and life on the road. Like the Wizard of Oz, I freely embrace being a bad wizard; I much prefer to be a good person. That feels more like home to me.

Lessons from the Big Chair: Chapter 2

- It does not help to act as though we are something we are not.
- The road that leads to change is fraught with danger and challenges for both you and your patients. Be brave; don't let fear stop you on the journey.
- Being of help to people who are learning to think and feel and act with courage will take you home.
- It's the journey that heals us; the journey is the solution. Embrace the road you're on.

Case Study: Martha

My first impression of Martha when I went to greet her in the waiting room was of a self-assured, engaging, sophisticated woman. She was a white woman in her mid-thirties, reading a novel she brought with her and clothed in a beautifully designed casual dress. Martha had a warm smile and a soft voice. A friend had recommended her to me for help coping with the end of a relationship. A romantic relationship of three years had ended abruptly for her when her fiancé declared that he no longer wanted to marry her and was planning to move a great distance away. As Martha began to tell me her story, I felt a strong affinity for what she was going through. I had a marriage end in much the same manner. She felt confused and devastated, unsure of what to do next in her life. I could certainly empathize with her anxiety and uncertainty.

For several sessions, we worked together processing what had happened and sharing a box of tissues. I had self-disclosed that I had a similar experience and understood the feeling of being shocked, lost, and abandoned. The fiancé had been the only boyfriend she had in the past decade. Along with Martha's grief, there was also an outpouring of fear and anger. "Why would he treat me this way?" "All he wanted was sex and I wasn't ready," "What is it about men that they think they can destroy me without any consequence?" The last two questions caught my attention and I asked if there had been other times in her life when she had had a similar experience of a man "just wanting sex" and "avoiding consequences for his behavior?" Something happened to Martha. She changed the subject rather quickly and I felt her withdraw from the emotional intimacy that we had established. I made a mental note to revisit my question in our next session.

The following week, I shared my observation of her discomfort the previous week and asked if I could reintroduce my question about any previous experiences of feeling "destroyed" by a man? I believe it's important to be respectful of reluctance on the part of a patient to respond to inquiries that may challenge their defenses. There's a reason they've built those walls. I also believe that it is our job as therapists to make it clear that we want to know what has hurt our patients; what unresolved, painful experiences they are carrying with them. We can't collude with patients to exclude important parts of their history; those significant past events that continue to shape them. While I don't want to crash through the wall, I do want to knock on the door.

Fortunately, Martha decided to let me in. When she was in her mid-twenties, she was brutally raped by a man she went out with. They were both in the same college class and it was their first "date." Martha had some previous boyfriends but was "saving myself for marriage" and had limited sexual experience. She had a very protected childhood in a loving, safe home and had never experienced a violent encounter with anyone. In the decade since the rape occurred, she never told anyone what had happened. I asked if she wanted to share more with me and she said she did, that she couldn't continue to hide how painful that event had been for her. Martha tried several times to tell me more details but simply became too overwhelmed to do so. She would begin the story of the rape and before she could get past the very beginning of the incident, she would break down in tears and stop.

When I asked what was getting in the way of sharing what happened, Martha told me that she was terribly fearful of what it would be like to share her experience with someone else. She had never talked about what happened and had done her best to forget it and just move on. The fear of how it would feel to invite that memory into her awareness and describe it to another person was overwhelming. She didn't know how to find the courage to tell me and to risk my being uncomfortable or judging her for not taking some action to report the incident. We talked through those concerns, but she remained too frightened to try and tell the story.

Several years prior to meeting Martha, I had attended an evening of innovative theater. One actor I remembered did a fascinating piece. He came on stage holding ten, 3x5 cards with a brief narrative written on each card. He explained to the audience that he was going to tell us a true story of something that happened to him, but it was up to us how the story would be told. The actor than flung the cards on the stage, turned them all down so the writing couldn't be seen, and asked audience members to come up on stage, pick up one of the cards, and hand it to him. A piece of his story was written on each of the cards. As he was handed a card by the audience member, he read what was on it. Although the story wasn't told in the order that it happened, everything came together by the end. The narrative was hardly linear, but it didn't need to be for us to understand what had happened. I thought it was a brilliant, creative way to tell a story. I hadn't thought about it until Martha was stuck trying to tell her story.

I wondered if telling her story in a nonlinear way might be helpful. It was clear that Martha was anticipating when the parts of the story were coming up that were most painful and shameful to her; the aspects that she feared revealing. I asked Martha if she could break down her story of the rape into at least 3 pieces: A beginning, a middle, and an end. I gave her a stack of 3x5 cards and invited her to use as many as she needed to write down exactly what had happened to her and to bring those to the next session. She was brave enough to agree to do so. It was an experiment to see if it would help her share what happened.

In the next session, I asked how the experiment had gone. Martha told me it had been a difficult week, but she had filled out nine of the cards and written the entire story on them. She shared that it was helpful to not have to do the whole thing at once; she was able to do at least a few cards every day. I asked her to shuffle the cards for a few minutes until she felt they were sufficiently reorganized. Then I had her lay them out on my desk. I told her I would pick up cards in the order that she pointed to them, hand the card to her, and ask her to read what was on it. If there was a card she didn't feel she could read by herself, I would help her if she asked. And so, her story was finally told.

There were tears and distress along the way, but she made it through. Her first statement after all the cards were read was how relieved she was that she could finally tell the truth. It was no longer a shameful secret that she carried with her, one that had affected her ability to be intimate with a man she loved. We celebrated her accomplishment and, in future sessions, were able to see how the secret had impacted her relationship with the fiancé. About two years after our work together ended, I received a wedding invitation from Martha. While I couldn't attend, I wrote to let her know how delighted I was for her and wished her a wonderful married life. Several years later, she sent me a photo of a happy looking trio; Martha, her husband Greg, and their newborn daughter, Sasha. I've kept that photo in my desk drawer at the office for many years.

Lesson from the Big Chair: Courage

My work with Martha was an experience I'll always remember. Her willingness to try something unusual, to "experiment" with me was such an act of courage for her. I was so appreciative of her willingness to take a risk and honored to be the one she trusted enough to tell. Those experiences of being the only person that a patient has disclosed a painful secret to are humbling. As we traveled that road together, I was grateful to be her companion. I learned a great deal from her about trust, determination, and courage. I also enjoyed the creativity of our work together. It was an experiment that we both undertook to see if discarding the linear narrative would work for her. Her success led me to use this idea with other trauma survivors and it has often proven helpful when they are telling their story. I learned from Martha that both patient and therapist must sometimes be brave enough to try something new.

3

THE PURSUIT OF HAPPINESS

The Nature of Unhappiness

It's certainly not unusual for us to seek psychotherapy because we are unhappy. We don't have the right job or partner or family. We've been treated badly or harmed by others. We feel that we can't get what we desire or deserve. Unhappiness is often created by the idea that we don't have something that we need: love, money, beauty, recognition, success. Most of us have an endless list of what we lack and what we should be doing to improve. We aren't smart enough, attractive enough, and wealthy enough.... we just aren't enough. "If happiness depends on the ratio of fulfilled desires to total desires, no person whose desires are infinite can be satisfied" (Pipher, 2016, p. 171). In fact, the need to constantly be doing something to improve yourself is a source of unhappiness (Seppala, 2016). We become human "doings" instead of human beings.

There's the sense that if we can arrive at a certain point somewhere in the uncertain future, we'll finally be happy. We put happiness on hold until we're thinner, finish our education, have a better job, find the right partner,

start a family, get the kids off to college, pay all our debts, are able to retire…
until we run out of time. We could always do better, but the sense that we
must delay satisfaction, peace of mind, or joy robs us of the happiness that
is here at this moment. Quite simply, if you're not happy now you're not as
likely to be happy later today, or tomorrow, or next year. As I'm writing this
book, when I find myself thinking about how happy I imagine I'll be when
it's published, I miss the pleasure of sitting quietly at my desk in my lovely
home, thinking about ideas that I find interesting and engaging in the creation of a book that I hope will be as useful to others who read it as it is to me
as I write it. There is pleasure in the moment that I don't want to miss.

Delusions About Happiness

Buddhist psychology focuses on several delusions that interfere with happiness. First, we suffer from the delusion that changing our circumstances is
the path to happiness. We believe that happiness is something that exists in
our relationships with other people or somewhere out in the world. What
we often find, however, is that the more we seek happiness as something
that exists in the trappings of our life, the more unhappy we become. Our
experience of feeling unhappy often begins with the thought that "If I
only…." then life would be good and I would be happy. It's the brass ring
that's just beyond our reach; that next house, next job, or next spouse. We
delude ourselves that happiness exists somewhere outside of our mind. The
belief that happiness is something that will come to us, rather than something that comes from us is guaranteed to generate unhappiness.

When I ask students, what would make them happy, they often say
"Winning the lottery." It's why we play the lottery; we love to fantasize
about how much better our lives would be if we won. While for most people, it's a harmless fantasy, in my work with problem gamblers I saw the
destruction that this delusional pursuit of happiness could inflict. In fact,
research shows that people who win a substantial amount of money through
gambling are ultimately as happy after the win as they were before (Dixon,
Nastally, & Waterman, 2010; Farrell, 2018; McCown & Chamberlain, 2000).
As a patient told me, "The only way to be happy after winning a jackpot is
to be happy before winning a jackpot." I have also worked with gamblers
who found that winning large jackpots made their lives much worse. They
no longer knew who to trust, they were suspicious of new relationships

("Do they like me or my money?") and family relationships often became much more problematic. One of the most common experiences in the early stages of a gambling disorder is a significant win which, like an intense high, makes the gambler just want more. It's a common diagnostic symptom in the history of compulsive gamblers. As one of my patients said, "I would certainly be happier if I had all the money I lost gambling".

Another delusion that creates unhappiness is the idea of permanence. When a patient tells me that they hate change and do their best to avoid it, I usually ask two things: "How good are you at avoiding change?" and "How happy are you?" "We can live wisely only when we accept the reality of change" (Kornfield, 2008, p. 231). When we encounter any experience or object that brings us joy, we want it to last forever. We try to hold tight to those people, things or experiences; to keep that moment alive through clinging to it. We want every kiss to be as exciting and romantic as the first one. Nothing, however, is permanent. It's unfailingly the case that trying to live outside of what is real will make us miserable. Buddhist practitioners deliberately contemplate the inevitability of change that is the nature of all things. It's a way to train our minds to appreciate what we have when it's a part of our life and to gracefully let it go when it's time is at an end.

For those who fear or avoid change, even the happiness of a moment disappears in the awareness that it will be gone. I see it in patients who, following a painful breakup, choose to remain alone in order to avoid suffering through that experience again. It's like refusing to eat because we understand we'll be hungry again later. When we are happy, it's as though we have a lovely visitor that we know will only be with us for a while, but when we are unhappy it seems as though a distressing invader has taken up permanent residence. It's always true that "this too shall pass," whether it's something pleasant or painful. It can be difficult to remember that unhappiness comes and goes, just as happiness does. What is now will not always be so.

Finally, unhappiness is rooted in forgetting who we are. When we feel ourselves as separate, alone in the world and dependent on some aspect of our identity, we are on the path to unhappiness. We are not our bodies, for even if our body is damaged or injured, we can feel whole. I like to remind myself that if all the space between the atoms in my body were somehow removed, I would be the size of a sugar cube. How can I be my body if it's mostly emptiness? We are not our mind, for our thoughts and different states of consciousness change continuously. Ideas, memories, bits of old songs, wondering what I'll have for dinner…my thoughts are not myself any more than a radio is music. Wisdom and my experience tell me that my sense of self is an illusion. I am not a separate entity. Who I am at this moment is not who I am in the next moment. We are so often caught up in our roles, our comedies and our dramas that we fail to recognize all beings share in a common life. Much of Buddhist practice is centered on relieving us of the delusion that we are beings separate from other beings. To explore that further, I recommend Jack Kornfield's book "The Wise Heart: A Guide to the Universal Teachings of Buddhist Psychology" (2008). For the past decade, I've read it continuously, starting it again as soon as I reach the end.

The Nature of Happiness

The question now becomes, what is happiness? The Dalai Lama describes that the purpose of our lives is to be happy (Lama, 2004). I like the idea that happiness is letting go of what you think your life is supposed to look like and embracing the life that you have. Happiness isn't getting what you want, it's wanting what you've got. It appears that "happiness stems not from how well things go but whether things go better than expected" (Gottleib, 2019, p. 133). We feel happy when our life fulfills our needs even though it might not fulfill all our wants. Happiness is a feeling of contentment that life is just as it should be. Those who are skilled at being happy learn to maintain that contentment even during difficult times. Focusing on what we don't have makes us miserable; appreciating what we do have makes us content. In other words, happiness comes when we have a state of mind in which we feel satisfied and fulfilled.

We tend to ask patients, "What makes you happy?" with the implication that there is someone or something outside of ourselves that we need in order to experience happiness. That question sets the expectation that happiness is dependent on getting something that we lack. I use terms such as "content," "satisfied," comfortable," or "at peace" rather than "happy" when thinking about what makes our lives good. I prefer to ask patients to tell me about times that they feel satisfied, that they are at peace with their life. I think of it that way for myself; how am I constructing happiness or unhappiness from my current circumstance or experiences? Happiness is a state of mind that is accessible despite our situation. If wealth or status, being thin enough or tall enough, having a shiny new car or a beautiful partner made us happy, then everyone who achieved those things would be happy and everyone who lacked those things would be miserable. It's easy to observe that this isn't so.

It's important to acknowledge that we live in a culture in the United States that seems to thrive on making us unhappy. Advertising, social media, and our fascination with beautiful celebrities guarantee that we will feel deprived and depressed. Comparing ourselves to others who are featured in movies or on the cover of magazines magnifies our anxieties about our bodies and our worth. Research has indicated that social media use increases feelings of depression and loneliness (Hunt, Marx, Lipson, & Young, 2018). Looking at people's photographs of exotic vacations and happy family events is a contrast to sitting in our home or office looking at a computer screen. It may seem as if everyone else is having a wonderful life while we look on in envy.

Learning Happiness

Becoming more at peace and satisfied in our life is something we learn. Fortunately, we have many guides and paths that we can follow. I have found Buddhist teachings helpful, but there are many ways to improve our experience of happiness. Some of us are fortunate to have families and teachers along the way that help build a foundation for satisfaction with our life. For most of us, however, it takes some effort and determination to seek out a philosophy and practice that we can follow. Luckily, we also have research that can provide some direction about how to create a happier life (Mongrain, Chin, & Shapira, 2011; Seligman, 2002; Watkins, McLaughlin, & Parker, 2019;). Two factors that most happy people have in common are gratitude and compassion. Those who appreciate what they have in life, even the parts that are challenging or painful, are happier people. Also, those who are of service to others, who practice compassion, are happier. Feeling that we have something to offer that can increase happiness in others is a direct road to our own happiness. To learn to be happy is to learn gratitude and compassion.

Gratitude

In Chapter 5, will explore the importance of developing compassion, so I will focus here on gratitude. If gratitude is important to well-being, it is useful to understand how that state of mind can be cultivated. To increase feelings of gratitude, one of my meditation practices is my grateful dish washing every evening. As a child, washing dishes was my least favorite chore. Now I look forward to washing the dishes after dinner. I first commit to being fully present as I wash dishes. I focus on each item as I clean it and think how fortunate I am to have eaten the food that was on the plate, how thankful I am to have what I need to buy, prepare, and serve healthy food. I thank about how much I appreciate all of the people who created the dish I'm rinsing; the people who designed it, who learned the skills to make it, all those who made it available for me to purchase, who built the store from where I bought it. That path of feeling gratitude for all the efforts of others to provide me with the food and dishes that I use goes on forever. I pay attention to wanting what I have. I am deeply thankful for all those who were kind enough to make a dish that I now enjoy using. It's a mindfulness practice that I often recommend to students and patients. Practicing gratitude is life-changing. It focuses our mind on what we have in our life rather than what we don't have. Instead of "The damned dishes are dirty again and need to be washed," it's "I'm so fortunate to have these dishes and the food that was on them."

I believe that for therapists, learning to create a grateful, positive mind is vital if we are to mature into the profession. Even regarding patients with whom I have not been able to connect or have a positive impact, I'm grateful that I had the chance to join them in their suffering for a while. At least they didn't suffer alone. I hope that they felt respected and accepted for our time together and that was helpful to them. For me, there was an opportunity to expand my capacity for compassion through my attempt to relate to them and understand their experience. Therapy sessions that don't go well always offer me an opportunity to develop a more grateful and compassionate mind.

The Pursuit of Happiness

There is a frustrating paradox that the act of pursuing happiness often makes us miserable. In fact, it can lead to worse circumstances if we don't appreciate the true nature of happiness. It's clear that if external circumstances secured a happy life, then the healthiest and wealthiest among us would be the happiest people on earth. Certainly, being healthy and having financial security are important for our quality of life. Having a comfortable life gives us safety and stability to focus on creating a happier mind. Being well and feeling secure is characterized by the absence of having to pay attention to how you're doing. Worries brought on by illness and financial insecurity or the pain of loss and trauma certainly challenge our sense of well-being and increase our stress. Even the happiest of people are unhappy in times of crisis. One thing I like to share with clients is that unhappiness is not an indicator of inadequacy or depression, it is a sign of intelligence. Ignorance is bliss.

Addiction as the Misguided Search for Happiness

Having worked for almost four decades in the substance abuse field, I've come to think of addiction as a misguided attempt at happiness. The "physics" of addiction is clear that what goes up must not only come down but will dig a much deeper hole than ever existed initially. Addiction is an escape plan that constructs its own prison. Below the surface of addiction, there is likely to be trauma. Gilbert (2019) at the Vinland National Center reports that 75% of women and men in substance abuse treatment report histories of abuse and trauma and 12%-34% of individuals report Post Traumatic Stress Disorder. The desire to mitigate the pain of a traumatic experience makes the use and misuse of mood-altering substances much more likely. The unfortunate truth is, drugs work. Psychoactive substances capture the brain by creating the illusion of relief or even ecstasy. Happiness, however, is not just relief from the suffering, it is a specific state of mind. Happiness that is not reliant on ingesting substances or unplanned, random, pleasant events or circumstances is constructed and maintained through being fully present in our lives. Addiction makes that impossible.

Any substance or activity that provides an illusion of happiness or numbs our unhappiness is likely to be addictive. "It is only through all manner of numbing compensations, distractions, and enchantments that we agree not to question the root cause of our troubles...But sooner or later, if we are not rendered totally insensitive, our defensive compensations begin to fail in their soothing and concealing purpose and, as a consequence, we begin to suffer" (Wilber, 1981). There is no more toxic, numbing compensation than addiction, whether it's to drugs, gambling, alcohol, sex, our phones, or any number of other pursuits that temporarily keep suffering at bay through creating an alternate reality. The catch is that our pain is guaranteed to lurk beneath our intoxication and grow stronger. When a substance or activity becomes our primary relationship in life, we will do hurtful things to ourselves and others. During addiction, any underlying trauma is fed by the increase of guilt, anger, fear, and despair until there is no room for happiness. What we try to avoid feeling feeds on our avoidance. That shadow of grief and misery, rage and regret are attached to us. Wherever we go, the pain goes too. Not feeling something doesn't mean it's not there.

I think of addiction as a journey away from the self. People become someone they never thought they could be – a liar, thief, child abuser, criminal. I believe that a person in the grip of addiction is a different person, much like Jekyll and Hyde. The idea of "in vino, veritas" (in wine is the truth) is a most unfortunate myth. People do not express their most deeply held feelings when under the influence of alcohol. In fact, it's the opposite. What is mistaken for an honest expression of feelings is the result of disinhibition in the frontal cortex, that part of the brain responsible for logic, reason, and the ability to monitor our thoughts and feelings. Difficult truths are only useful if they're infused with compassion and intoxication makes that impossible. We become more primal, not more truthful.

I'm delighted by the addiction treatment fields embrace of mindfulness training. Meditation practice has been a cornerstone of my life for 50 years and is largely responsible for helping me both manage distress and expand happiness in my daily experience. Learning to stay present in our life, regardless of the circumstances, is the essence of mindfulness. Those beginning recovery from addiction often wake up to a mountain of pain, guilt, sadness, and anger. Everything is a mess. The life that they left when the addiction took hold is there waiting with its companion; the time that they lost while being addicted. It's an amazingly difficult awakening. Mindfulness provides a means of staying in that painful place without being overwhelmed and retreating. It allows us to accept our experience rather than avoid it. Mindfulness creates the path for the journey back to the real self that was held hostage by addiction.

Early in sobriety, people find they are capable of both pain and pleasure again. An experience that I really cherish is seeing someone in recovery have the first, tentative experience of joy. Just waking up and not feeling sick, being able to enjoy a joke, playing music, or making a painting.

They have a return of the happiness of small things and the capacity for being present in their life again. Learning how to be in our own skin and to celebrate the unfolding of our life feels miraculous when it has been absent during periods of addiction. It's such a gift to just enjoy our own company and that of others.

The Difference Between Pain and Suffering

We all have pain in our lives, but why do some people suffer more than others? Everyone experiences illness and loss. Everyone gets their share of hurt. "Most of the craziness in the world – violence, addictions, and frenetic activity – comes from running from pain" (Pipher, 2016, p. 54). While we can't avoid pain, how much we suffer is under our control. It's what we tell ourselves about our painful experiences that determine our level of suffering. If someone I love doesn't love me that is painful. If, however, I tell myself that I am unlovable or that this person was "the one" and I'll never love or be loved again, I am creating suffering. Pain happens to us, suffering is largely self-inflicted.

I often spend time with clients exploring the difference between pain and suffering so that they can better manage the damage created by an unrealistic or catastrophic evaluation of painful experiences. Learning to manage our internal dialogue regarding misfortune is a skill worth developing. I'm grateful for the research and techniques that are the foundation of cognitive therapy and for applications of mindfulness practice to increase our skills in coping with problems. Both have made our work as therapists so much more effective and have been personally helpful. It's difficult for any of us to embrace pain and distress as useful, but it is almost always what motivates us to make changes and accept challenges that can lead us to a greater satisfaction and bring joy into our lives.

Many of us who seek therapy or become therapists have a history of trauma: child abuse, domestic violence, abandonment, illness, and loss. Sadly, it's too late to have a happy past. It is not too late, however, to create a happier life from this point forward. It is hard work to encourage people to let themselves off the hook for experiences that were beyond their control. It can be useful to review the circumstances of the traumatic events and determine if any changes might help prevent a future occurrence, such as carrying an alarm or having an evacuation plan for severe weather. If there are things that can be done to mitigate similar future traumas, do them. Many times, however, the experience was unavoidable and unpreventable.

Guilt is an especially challenging type of suffering because it helps to maintain an illusion that we could have controlled an uncontrollable situation. Guilt is a judgment we pass on ourselves for something that we probably had little or no power to prevent or avoid. For survivors of rape, combat situations, and other traumatic events, it's not unusual to cling to the fantasy that the experience could have been avoided or mitigated if only we had done something different. It's a way of trying to claim responsibility for something done to us, not by us. It provides a small hope that if we only change that one thing that we did before the traumatic event, it would not have happened to us. If only… The reality is, we did the best we could to survive or cope. I sometimes ask patients, "If you lived in a culture that didn't have any conception of 'guilt,' what do you think you would be feeling instead"? Often, that allows survivors to acknowledge the anger, fear, and grief about being harmed by an experience they couldn't escape.

Whereas guilt is the feeling that we *are* something bad, remorse is the acknowledgment that we've *done* something bad. Remorse is a recognition of something that we did, either intentionally or unintentionally, that harmed ourselves and others. When we are responsible for an action that created harm, there is the opportunity to make amends and do what we can to correct the situation. Making amends, whether to ourselves or others, allows us to accept responsibility and repair the damage to the extent possible. In 12 Step programs, the ninth step instructs people to "Make direct amends…whenever possible, except when to do so would injure them or others." (Bill, 1976). There are times when acknowledging how we have harmed someone else is important in helping us to feel more at peace with ourselves.

Making amends is more than an apology, it is taking action to repair the damage. For example, if I kicked your door down in a fit of anger and later said "I'm sorry," that's an apology but not an amend. An amend is when I bring my tools and fix the door. I would avoid doing more harm by *not* saying "I only kicked your door down because I was upset when your husband refused to divorce you during our affair." An amend is also a commitment to not inflict more harm. Making amends lets us practice compassion through doing what we can to repair the damage done to someone we hurt. It's a good way to make room for greater peace of mind and happiness.

Happiness and Suffering

Buddhist philosophy focuses on the dilemma of happiness and suffering. The goal of Buddhist practice is to attain enlightenment which is an end to suffering.

> "Everybody wants to be happy. Everybody wants to be loved and accepted as they are. Everybody wants to feel clear and strong and loving in their turn. Everybody wants to live in a happy and peaceful world. Everybody wants enough food. Everybody wants to be free from pain. Understanding what we all want is not difficult. It is how to get there that is the problem" (Claxton, 1990, p. 34).

The treasure buried in unhappiness is how often it is the foundation for change and transformation. Being sick and tired of being sick and tired can be highly motivational. One of the gifts of therapy is the opportunity to help others transform suffering into connection, compassion, and wisdom. The chaos of a crisis can give birth to a greater sense of freedom and empathy, a stronger awareness that each of us face suffering, and that we can support and comfort each other. People who have grown through their experience of suffering are often more compassionate and understanding toward others who continue to suffer. In 12 Step groups, the 12th step asks us to use what we've learned in our own recovery to reach out to others who are still addicted. It's through building compassion that we build happiness.

NOTES FROM THE BIG CHAIR

Fortunately, in the past decade, the study of happiness has helped provided insights that are important for therapists to understand, both for the benefit of our patients and ourselves. Those of us in the big chair have a responsibility to learn what creates a happy life so that we can bring that experience to our work with others. If we are to help our patients, we need to know what the research on happiness tells us about how to increase our sense of life satisfaction and peace of mind. We must be able to lessen our own suffering if we are to guide others through theirs. It's hard to find our way out of the darkness if we haven't lit our own candle. Gretchen Rubin spent a year dedicating herself to becoming happier and her book, *The Happiness Project* (2009) is a lovely guide to build a more meaningful and happier life. The challenges are not easy, but her experience validates much of the research and philosophy of what makes for a happy life. One of her "splendid truths"

---

is that: "One of the best ways to make yourself happy is to make other people happy; one of the best ways to make other people happy is to be happy yourself." (Rubin, 2009, p. 316).

When students start their training to become therapists, I congratulate them on making a career choice that is likely to increase their happiness. One thing we know about happiness is that being of service to others is a meaningful endeavor that increases our sense of contentment. Despite the challenges inherent in this work, those of us who stay with it tend to be a pretty satisfied group. We fall between bank tellers and bus drivers on career satisfaction scales (National Opinion Research Center) which is somewhere around the 60th percentile on the job happiness scale. Other chapters of this book explore some of the challenges of the profession: burnout, traumatic contagion, work overload, stressful patients, compassion fatigue, and other factors. Doing this work and maintaining a happy life isn't always easy.

To inform my work on this book, I've been reading other writers, all of whom have spent decades practicing psychotherapy. I am struck by the consistent themes of being grateful and happy to have a life in the big chair.

- "...there is no better work than the work we do" (Pipher, 2016, p. 180).
- "I like the feeling that I am always working, always thinking, and always trying to make sense of what is happening. And yet I am never working because even time spent with clients helps me learn more about the world and myself" (Kottler, 2017, p. 50).
- "As much as I may have helped my clients on their journey to healing, I received far more than I gave" (Bugaeff, 2018, Preface).
- "There is extraordinary privilege here. And extraordinary satisfaction, too" (Yalom, 2017, p. 256).
- "Psychotherapy is a profoundly optimistic endeavor and our optimism is one of our most important contributions to the therapeutic relationship" (Cozolino, 2004, p. 208).

Happiness is not something that just happens; we create it daily. We take care of ourselves and can say "yes" or "no" when we need to. We are grateful for our chance to be alive. We connect to others and learn how to love, we recognize and enjoy the grace of small kindnesses and simple pleasures. Mindfulness helps us stay in the moment which is the only place where happiness resides.

Lessons from the Big Chair: Chapter 3

- Happiness isn't getting what we want, it's wanting what we have.
- Happiness doesn't come to you, it comes from you.
- Gratitude, compassion, and service to others are pathways to increase happiness.
- Suffering is often the door to making positive changes.
- Painful experiences are unavoidable, but we can determine how much we suffer.

A Story

A wise person was asked to explain the difference between suffering and happiness. This was their reply:

"Imagine that you are in a large banquet hall with hundreds of other people around an enormous table. All of you are starving to death. The table is laden to overflowing with all the most wonderful food you can imagine; everything that your heart desires is there for you. The only problem is that all the utensils you must use to eat with are three feet long. Try as you might, you can't feed yourself with them, they are simply too long. Everyone at the table continues to starve. That is suffering.

Now, imagine that you are in a large banquet hall with hundreds of other people around an enormous table. All of you are starving to death. The table is laden to overflowing with all the most wonderful food you can imagine; everything that your heart desires is there for you. The only problem is that all the utensils you must use to eat with are three feet long. And so, you use them to feed each other. That is happiness."

4

NO MATTER WHERE YOU GO, THERE YOU ARE

Never a Boring Day

One of my favorite things about being a psychotherapist is that I've never had a boring day in more than 40 years. I've had times that were filled with sadness and pain when a client attempted suicide and other times overflowing with joy and gratitude when a client was finally able to break free of an abusive relationship. There are days when it feels like the big chair is a seat on a roller coaster. From one session to the next, I may give a standing ovation to a client who, after years of addiction to narcotics got their one-year sober chip and in the next session, reach for my own box of tissues when a client finally talks about his abuse as a child. It's still amazing to me that people are willing to trust me with the most hurt and vulnerable parts of themselves; to share in therapy what they may never have told anyone else. I am in awe of people's determination to be better and I'm honored when someone gives me the opportunity to bear witness to their experience. "Often the therapist is the only audience viewing great dramas and acts of courage" (Yalom, 2017, p. 14). Sharing in the struggles and accomplishments of so many people is a transformative experience. Clients are not the only ones who are changed by being in therapy.

Many of us start our career in the big chair thinking we are the Wizard; some never make the transformation to being Dorothy (see Chapter 2). Being humble is a useful attitude to develop. The biggest complaint I hear from patients who have left therapy with other practitioners is that "they seemed to know who I was and what I needed before they even met me." Humility and uncertainty are virtues in this profession. It is humbling to be a companion on a patient's journey through the most frightening, confusing, overwhelming parts of their lives and to observe their resilience and strength. I often wonder if I would have been able to survive some of the experiences that clients describe, and I sometimes share that observation with them. To me, it is a gift to be invited along as a companion through those parts of another's life and to observe how telling our story begins to change us. I have come to believe that an integral part of how therapy works is that changing our stories changes us.

Challenges

There are numerous challenges that we must learn to cope with as therapists. When I warn students how hard this work can be, I'm really commenting on the effects of being emotionally intimate with patients in crisis. Traumatic contagion is part of being human. Our brains are activated by seeing or hearing about someone else's trauma in the same way as if it was happening to us (Cozolino, 2004). Working with trauma in psychotherapy is itself traumatic. We now recognize that working in the helping professions has a profound effect on us, whether through direct exposure to trauma (first responders, emergency room staff) or through secondary exposure when we listen to our patients share their histories of victimization, abuse, or other trauma (Mathieu, 2012). Compassion fatigue, vicarious trauma, secondary trauma, and burnout are all possible effects of the work we do as psychotherapists. Mathieu (2012) defines them as follows:

Compassion fatigue refers to the profound emotional and physical erosion that takes place when helpers are unable to refuel and regenerate.
Vicarious trauma describes the transformation of our view of the world due to the cumulative exposure to traumatic images and stories. This is

accompanied by intrusive thoughts and imagery and difficulty ridding ourselves of the traumatic experiences recounted by our clients.

Secondary traumatic stress (STS) is the result of bearing witness to a traumatic event (or to a series of events), which can lead to PTSD-like symptoms.

Burnout has to do with the stress and frustration caused by the workplace: Having poor pay, unrealistic demands, heavy workload, heavy shifts, poor management, and inadequate supervision. (p. 14).

For many of us, a therapist is the only person who is willing to let us really express our suffering without the fear of being judged. When we let patients know they can share anything that is troubling them with us, be prepared! Even four decades into my career, I still find myself wishing I hadn't heard something that a patient just told me. There are often good reasons that we don't share certain experiences with anyone other than a professional person; we have shocking, shameful, traumatic events that are hiding in us as toxic secrets. Hearing those is a truly difficult task for those of us in the big chair. I find it important to keep myself in the present moment and maintain my awareness that this person is now safely in my office, having survived that experience and working to cope more effectively with what happened to them.

I believe that people who come into this profession burn out early because they are still learning to be an effective therapist. It's rare that I hear my colleagues talk to trainees about how hard occupying the big chair can be. We risk our own emotional well-being when we engage intimately with others who are in emotional turmoil. When we occupy the big chair, we are constantly reminded of our own wounds. Other's pain connects us to our own. Humans are hard wired to identify with each other's vulnerabilities; if we weren't, horror movies would have no effect on us. If we are to engage empathically, we can't retreat into our own defenses. We offer our vulnerability and courage in order to encourage patients to do the same.

Stay in the Chair – Be Patient with Patients

Jumping to conclusions about who a patient is, what they are experiencing and what they need is common when we are learning to sit in the big chair. I remember being very anxious and excited when I started seeing patients;

anxious to figure them out as quickly as possible so I could move on to giving advice and solving their problems. Essentially, when we do this, we are taking care of our own anxiety at the expense of the client. We are treating them like a problem instead of a person. I think of it as the Pepe LePew dilemma. In the classic Looney Tunes cartoons, Pepe LePew was an amorous French skunk who falls in love with what he thinks is a charming female skunk. The object of his affections is, however, a black cat who has walked under a paintbrush with white paint on it and then fallen into a vat of stinky cheese. Every episode is *exactly* the same. The dilemma is thinking we are seeing something that we are not. An old diagnostic trope is that if it looks like a skunk, smells like a skunk, and walks like a skunk, it's probably a skunk. That's usually true, except when it's not. Try to avoid the Pepe LePew dilemma – you may be seeing an unfortunate black cat rather than a skunk. Be patient, gather more information, and don't become too enamored of your first impressions.

It can be terrifying, especially in the beginning, to be in close connection to someone who is deeply depressed, who was abused, who is hostile and defensive. Just like the patient, we are vulnerable emotionally. It is difficult to be close to someone who is suffering and not want to be the Wizard with a magic formula to end their misery. Our natural tendency is to throw suggestions at someone until we come up with one that fixes them. One of my training exercises with students is to practice initial interviews with each other. They have 45 minutes to listen to their "patient," but the patient is instructed to immediately end the interview if the therapist offers them a suggestion. If they hear "Have you...," the patient stands up, ends the session, and makes a note of how long the interview lasted. Most dyads don't make it to the full 45 minutes; some end rather abruptly in the first 5 minutes. Offering suggestions is a way to protect ourselves by diverting a patient from their narrative, a narrative that is sometimes very uncomfortable to hear. It's a natural defense; we don't want to be traumatized by connecting to someone else's trauma.

The best advice I ever had from a supervisor was "Don't just do something, sit there." Be present, be patient, be perceptive, and realize that's the hardest thing to do. It's difficult to help new colleagues learn that, "our job is not to provide immediate relief to clients or banish their pain, but rather to allow them to wallow in self-pity until such time that they feel sufficient commitment and motivation to do the hard work involved"

(Kottler & Carlson, 2014, p. 138). We often need time to vent, share our outrage or despair, or just feel hurt and be comforted that someone will hear us. Our greatest skill is our presence. Stay with the patient and their narrative until they are ready to let it go and move on.

Patients are not broken, so we don't need to rush to fix them. Experience has helped me be more patient and curious, more willing to be surprised instead of making assumptions. I love having my first impressions of a patient shattered as I get to know them and learn more about their story. I find that practicing this compassionate curiosity as a professional has also made my life outside the office less frustrating and annoying. It's easier now to appreciate that the person who cuts me off in traffic or the student who falls asleep in class has a story that I don't know, one that may be shaping their actions at any given time.

Be the Duck

I describe this experience of being fully present with a patient in crisis as "being the duck." At the aquarium in Tampa where I live, there is a wonderful exhibit with fish and ducks where you can see both above and below the water. I'm always struck by how calm a duck appears on the surface while its feet may be a flurry of movement. Being a therapist is often like that: I appear calm on the surface, but underneath I'm thinking "Oh CRAP!" "WHAT THE HELL?" Don't panic. Over time, you learn to be the duck. Even so, there will be times when you'll wish you'd studied accounting instead; when you just want to get up from the big chair and walk out of the office because of how sad, frightened, or angry you are about what you've heard.

Staying calm on the surface is a skill that takes time to master and all experienced therapists have their unique strategies. When our patients are at their worst, we must be at our best. When I feel particularly provoked or shocked by something a patient is saying, I revert to my "meeting a bear in the woods" strategy I learned when hiking in Colorado. Be still, keep breathing, don't make any noise, and don't run. I keep focused on the patient, check my facial expressions (I tend to frown when I hear something challenging), lean in a bit (so the patient knows they haven't scared me off), and do my best to stay connected. When a patient is sharing something that feels embarrassing or shameful, they often look away, but I want to be sure I don't so when they look back at me, I'm there. As Kottler (2017) reminds us, "You will see people when they are at their worst, and you will be expected to present yourself at your best. Every time." (p. 81).

Those who are planning a career in this field need to reflect on their willingness to take on the role of witness and companion to deeply hurt and disturbed patients, given the emotional toll it can take. As Kottler (2017) notes, "…we listen to stories that are so extraordinary, so heart wrenching that they are sometimes beyond what we can possibly hold." (p. 71). We don't talk enough with our students and trainees about what it means to sit with someone else's pain and to hold their stories and secrets. No one stays in this profession for very long without encountering a patient whose story haunts them. Most of us who have been in the big chair for decades have an encyclopedia of horror stories that we carry with us. We are repositories of hurtful secrets that may never have been shared with anyone else. Just as we desire relief from pain and suffering for our patients, we also must learn to transform outrage and despair into compassion and hope. The most important experience for patients is to be met with respect, caring and understanding.

Becoming Competent

This is a profession that people mature into if they can persevere and learn from their relationships with patients. Despite our best efforts as educators, we can't really prepare students for what will happen when they begin to occupy the big chair. Competence takes time to develop in this profession. One of the aspects of being a therapist that I enjoy is the rewards for maturity. Being a 68-year-old female renders me invisible in some social situations, but not as an occupant of the big chair. In this profession, maturity and longevity are respected and generally seen as positive. When I was beginning my career and watching senior clinicians conducting sessions, it seemed magical to me that they could be so unshakeable, so skilled at both guiding and following their patients. I had a clear appreciation of how my sessions seemed to proceed – like driving on a bumpy road with lots of detours – and how their sessions seemed so purposeful and focused like a smooth stretch of highway. Master therapists learn from the most important teachers, their patients. As Jon Carlson notes, "Although I have learned some important things from research studies, conferences, workshops, and even books…most of my best supervisors and teachers have been my clients" (Kottler & Carlson, 2014, p. 7). Becoming a competent psychotherapist takes time, effort, humility, and appreciation that we truly learn how to be a therapist by being with those who seek our help.

There's a progression of competence that I like to share with students. First, you're an Unconscious Incompetent. You don't know much, and you don't know you don't know. As you get through your first few sessions and find yourself at a loss for words or with a patient who is frustrated with you for annoying them with suggestions of things they've already thought about, you become a Conscious Incompetent. You begin to realize how little you know and how much there is to learn. If you then devote yourself to learning, practicing, self-awareness, and patiently listening to your patients, over time you become an Unconscious Competent. Through supervision and experience, you begin to have some success but aren't yet sure what you're doing that works. Finally (for me it was about a decade into my career), you become a Conscious Competent. You are more aware of what is helpful and what isn't and begin to understand your unique strengths and talents. You learn how to be effective in the big chair only through experience; there are no shortcuts. We also cycle through that progression repeatedly during our careers. I had developed some competence at treating mental health issues during my first decade working at a state hospital and a community mental health center. When I began working in addiction treatment, the competence progression started over again as I was learning about that specific issue and population.

Several interpersonal traits that help build competence in this profession are humility, curiosity, patience, compassion, and a bit of masochism. "What other occupation has built into it the frustration of feeling helpless, stupid, and lost as a necessary part of the work?" (Ghent, 1999, p. 236). We must learn to build our skills on that foundation and accept the repeated experiences of confusion, helplessness, and uncertainty that we are subjected to in the process of building competence. Therapists who are not self-aware enough to recognize, accept, and learn from those experiences are at best incompetent and at worst dangerous.

Psychotherapist, Know Thyself

It's almost inevitable that I have at least one patient I'm seeing who is struggling with something that is familiar to me. It can be so tempting to stop them in mid-sentence and say, "You think YOUR boss is an idiot, let me tell you...." It's a unique requirement of therapists that we engage in continuous exploration of our biases, family experiences, relationships, reactions to clients, mental health, and happiness. While I prefer a congenial, collaborative relationship with a surgeon or dentist, their ability to help me isn't compromised if they behave like an arrogant asshole. They can do a good job regardless of their personality traits. Not so with therapists. Instead of using scalpels or drills, we depend on ourselves. "Everything we therapists do or say or feel as we sit with our patients is mediated by our histories; everything I've experienced will influence how I am in any given session..." (Gottlieb, 2019, p. 114). If we are hoping to guide our patients to a better understanding and acceptance of the parts of themselves that are difficult to acknowledge, we need to be willing to acknowledge and work on those parts of ourselves. Master therapists are often able to work beyond technique or theory to "use their distinctly personal characteristics to empower their helping efforts" (Kottler & Carlson, 2014, p. 167). Socrates said that "To know thyself is the beginning of wisdom."

Being a psychotherapist requires that we treat ourselves with the same degree of empathy and compassion that we extend to our clients. Therapists who are not on good terms with themselves or who ignore their own dilemmas are loose cannons. A supervisor once told me that "No one you work with can get better than you are." She didn't mean that I had to have a perfect, pain-free life, just that I couldn't get away with ignoring my own needs and concerns (see Chapter 7). If I am unaware of myself in the therapy relationship, I can't be of help to others and, in fact, could do more harm than good. If I am feeling lonely and unloved, it becomes a temptation to seek companionship and romance through my patients. I must constantly and consistently work on my own concerns outside the therapy relationship with patients or I risk manipulating or even abusing patients to meet my own needs. I always appreciate the reminder when I'm flying that if there is an emergency, I must put on my oxygen mask first if I'm to help others put on theirs. When I neglect my own well-being, I potentially put others at risk.

Learning to Dance

Learning to attend to the process of therapy is a difficult skill to teach in a classroom and, I believe, even more difficult to teach online. As the COVID-19 pandemic has closed our college classrooms, I'm struggling to teach certain classes like "Basic Counseling Skills." So much of communication is nonverbal and there are so many subtle signals of our attentiveness that are off the screen. What's on the screen, usually a talking head, is magnified and becomes the singular target that we focus on for nonverbal feedback. A downward glance that would have been unimportant in a face to face meeting suddenly is a sign of disinterest or rejection. I'm not very skilled at using technology as an intermediary and still trying to learn how to dance with screens in the middle of the relationship.

Learning to be present in the immediacy of a psychotherapy session is rather like learning to dance. You can watch others dance, review charts showing the steps for the dance, and talk with people who are experienced dancers, but until you get on the dance floor with someone else in your arms and the music starts, you don't know how to dance. You understand the content of a dance, the steps and rhythms, but not the process. The process takes place in the immediacy of the relationship. Content is much easier to dissect and track in a session, but the content is embedded in the process. In fact, the process determines the content.

When I watch videos of a trainee in session with a patient, I sometimes turn off the sound and the trainee and I will just watch the dance. Who is speaking more often? Does the therapist look connected? Bored? Nervous? How does the patient look? Are they engaged when the therapist is speaking? As the session progresses, are they becoming better dance partners? Is there a rhythm to how they interact that seems to connect them? It's helpful to look beyond content to watch the connection as it builds or disintegrates. When that connection seems fragile, we turn on the sound and listen to what's happening. That often gives us a way to explore transference and countertransference, to further explore what seemed to be a challenge in the session. Likewise, when I see the therapist and patient lean in or mirror an emotional reaction in an empathic way, we turn on the sound to see what the content tells us was bringing them together. It's an interesting way to really look at the dance steps the therapist is engaged in with the patient.

A session with a patient and therapist who have established a good therapeutic relationship is very different than their first interview. The content being shared has greater depth; there's a flow between the therapist and patient. We are learning how to dance together, getting a better sense of the timing and give and take that makes for a stronger connection. With effective therapists, they know how to adjust their reactions to fit the patient's style. Different partners dance differently, some like a slow dance, some need time to rest between songs, and some will run you ragged all over the dance floor. It's the patient who determines the type of dance you do, but it's the therapist's job to take the lead. The therapist guides the patient, encourages them to take new steps, acknowledges their skillful moves, and challenges their missteps.

We Bring Who We Are

No one is free of biases, opinions, prejudices, or cultural influences. The idea that we are neutral observers is a delusion. By the time we reach adulthood, we have accumulated a Pandora's Box of preconceptions and partisan notions. How we bring who we are to the therapy room makes a difference. Patients who have seen different therapists bring the same story with them, but their relationship with each therapist determines how the story unfolds and where it leads. I'm pretty sure that most students who were in training during the mid-1960s and 1970s watched the film in which Carl Rogers, Fritz Perls, and Albert Ellis each demonstrated their approach to psychotherapy by interviewing Gloria (Three approaches to psychotherapy, 1965). The film is a historical document now, but it's a good example of the influence of the therapist in determining the behavior of the patient. Although Gloria's story is the same, what moves to the foreground or background of the narrative is very different based on the therapist with whom she is speaking. When I first watched it in graduate school, I was focused on the content of what she shared. Now, I'm much more focused on how she related differently to each of the therapists, how each of them brought out a unique aspect of her personality and narrative.

Many who come to this profession have a history of trauma, family problems, addiction and other experiences that create the lens through which we evaluate our relationships. We see the world not as it is, we see the world as we are. If we ignore those influences and how they guide us, it's like a surgeon with a rusted scalpel or dentist with a blunt drill. I grew up with a mother who was prejudiced toward people of color. When I was a sophomore in high school in Texas in the late 1960s, the public schools became integrated. What that meant was a group of about 15 African-American high school students was bused in from their neighborhood to our white suburb and our all white high school of more than two thousand students. The first day they were there, I talked at dinner that night about seeing several of them in the hallway between classes. My mother told me "Be polite, but don't invite any of them to our home." It wasn't until I was in college that I met and established friendships with people who weren't white. I continue to work to understand how my family's priviledged legacy impacts my relationships and challenges me. I've had very generous and kind colleagues, students, and patients of color who have helped me appreciate what I represent to them as a white woman. I'm grateful for their patience and guidance.

I understand that I represent something to those I work with. For some, I'm the kindly, warm-hearted grandmother who protected them when their parents were fighting. For some, I'm a privileged, old white woman who grew up in a middle-class white suburb with parents who could afford to send me to college. For others, I'm an idiot who is a waste of their time and money, but they must see me because someone else made them go. I'm a different therapist with every person I see. An important part of making a therapeutic connection is to determine who I represent to my patient and what their expectations are of how I will treat them. Knowing what I represent helps me to both connect to the patient and to challenge them. Even loving grandmothers can hold you accountable for your choices and idiot's can care about your well-being. I think of it as being a coherent chameleon; I'm always who I am, but I change in response to what others may need from me.

Life Away from the Big Chair

I think it's important to consider some of the dilemmas that therapists encounter outside of the office when they're sitting at home on the sofa instead of in the big chair. Engaging with patients on a very intimate level can be exhilarating but is also exhausting. It's not unusual after a particularly challenging day at the office for me to want to come home and just sit on the sofa and binge watch Netflix. I'm mentally tired and just want to do something mindless. Being "on" all day means I want to be "off" for a few hours. That doesn't mean, however, that family or friends don't need me to be there with them. There are chores to be done, bills to pay, meals to cook, and all the daily tasks that demand our attention. For those with children, it's time for the second shift to begin. While being needed is gratifying, it can be draining.

It's also difficult to come home at the end of a challenging day and know that I can't really share what's happened. I have a responsibility to protect patient confidentiality and besides, my partner doesn't really want to know which is wise on his part. Psychotherapists, police, and attorneys share that hardship. Those outside the profession can't really appreciate how demanding the work can be, especially when I hear or see something that has an enormous emotional impact on me. Although I've learned over the years to leave the work in the office, I periodically see a patient who really affects me, someone who triggers a feeling of helplessness, anger, or despair. There are some days that I take a short walk to catch my breath before I head home. "Despair is part of what we do; it may even be an asset to our work when transformed to heighten our empathic powers" (Kottler & Carlson, 2014, p. 250). I need time on those days to reconnect with my belief in the possibility of transformation and to remind myself of the impermanence of all things.

Being a therapist can also mean that we want to step in and help in our personal relationships when our help may not be needed or wanted. Most of us have experienced someone we love telling us to "Stop being a therapist"! The nature of our work "…means enjoying intimacy without the loss of control that intimacy usually requires" (Kottler, 2017, p. 2). Supporting a patient in confronting someone they love but have a problem with is vastly different than me telling someone I love, "We need to talk." We get used to being listened to with respect and deference, something that isn't likely to happen in our personal relationships. It's easy to become convinced that we are "special" because we are often treated that way by patients and students. Fortunately, I'm not very good at convincing those I've been in social or intimate relationships with just how special I am. Our loved ones know us for the fallible, unreasonable, ridiculous people we often are. They've seen behind the smoke and mirrors and know full well that the Wizard is just another insecure, imperfect human being. It's a challenge to not see ourselves as the Wizard when we've had transformative, intense, inspiring experiences with our patients; experiences that changed their lives and ours. I'm aware that I like being needed and asked for my thoughts or advice. Having others treat you as though you have some power to fix broken things in their life is seductive. That's a type of respect and acknowledgment that can be addictive, even though I know it's based on false assumptions. It's hard sometimes to go from the big chair to the living room sofa and step away from that role.

We work with patients in a rule-bound, time-limited context with a focus on their needs and goals. At home, the effects of that professional discipline can make me long to be the center of attention; to be self-indulgent and insensitive to loved ones. I sometimes hear that voice in the back of my mind yelling "What about ME!" As is true for others, I need time to vent, to share my outrage or frustration, or to just feel hurt and be comforted that someone will hear me. There's a longing that I feel occasionally to just have a respite from the responsibilities I carry and the secrets I hold; a wish to have someone carry me off for a long weekend at the beach. I'm so appreciative when a friend or colleague asks me "How are you doing?" and just listens for a while to all the typical joys and sorrows that make up my life. Psychotherapy is not a good career choice for loners or stoics. We need others in our life who remind us to just be a human being; who love us for who we are rather than what we do. Therapists face the same challenges as everyone else. I want to be a good partner and friend, an active member of my neighborhood and community. I want to have fun, see the world, be with those I love when they're hurting and need to be comforted. I want to love and be loved, to be happy and sad, and to learn to live a good life. Fortunately, the more I engage in making my life interesting, loving, and worthwhile, the more I bring to my work in the big chair.

Lessons from the Big Chair: Chapter 4

- Sharing in the struggles and accomplishments of so many people is a transformative experience.
- Hearing the traumatic, toxic secrets of others is a truly difficult task.
- Try to avoid the Pepe LePew dilemma – you may be seeing an unfortunate black cat rather than a skunk.
- Don't just do something, sit there. Be present, be patient, be perceptive.
- We need to remember to put on our own oxygen mask first before we help others.
- We see the world not as it is, we see the world as we are.
- Who you are represents something to every patient you encounter.
- Having others treat you as though you have some power to fix broken things in their life is seductive.

Case Study: Luis

Luis was referred to our community mental health center in San Angelo, Texas by his 3rd grade teacher who was concerned that he might be exhibiting signs of a serious mental disorder. When his mother and father brought him to our center, I was immediately charmed by what an intelligent, engaging 9-year-old boy he was. Luis came into the office with his parents both as a patient and as the interpreter; neither of his parents spoke English with any fluency. It was clear that Luis was used to assisting his parents in navigating through the challenges that are part of being in a country where you don't speak the language.

I first asked them to tell me about the family and provide some history. The family had moved from a small, very poor village in Mexico to the United States when Luis was 6 years old so that both he and his older sister could get a better education and his parents could find work. Their father's mother, Inez, had moved to Texas with them and had passed away from stomach cancer two months earlier. It was clear from their reactions that Inez's death was very difficult for them to talk about. She was the matriarch of the family and much beloved. I asked them to tell me a favorite story about her and Luis talked about her love of cooking and how he had tried to learn to make tortillas from her but could never make them as round and flat as she did.

After getting acquainted, I asked what had brought them to see me? Luis's mother had gotten a call from his teacher the previous week. The teacher, Ms. Childress, was concerned about some drawings that Luis was making and stories that he was telling the other children. Ms. Childress sent home several drawings that Luis had made of his grandmother and they brought them to the session to share with me. I asked Luis to tell me about the drawings. All of them depicted Inez at different places in their home; seated in a chair in Luis's room, joining the family at dinner, looking on as Luis and his sister Dolores did their homework at the kitchen table. As he described them, Luis used the present tense: "Here is grandmother sitting in my room last night talking with me," "This is grandmother bringing dinner to the table for Dolores's 12th birthday last week," "Grandmother helps my sister and me do our homework every evening." It was this description that

Ms. Childress had found so disconcerting. When she had asked Luis about his grandmother's death and how she could still be doing all those things, Luis had insisted that she was still there and that he always looked forward to talking with her before bed, just as he always had.

I finished the intake and asked if the family would come back the following week. In gathering other information, there were no "red flags" regarding a serious mental disorder, but Luis's insistence that he still interacted with his grandmother was puzzling. Like his teacher, I was worried about whether this was a sign of a delusional process or some denial of the reality of the grandmother's death. I was fortunate to have a supervisor, Dr. Carlos Hernandez, who was raised in Mexico, fluent in Spanish and, when I described Luis and my concerns, he was eager to join us for the next session. He told me "I think I know what might be happening but let me talk directly with the parents to see if my hypothesis is right."

When the family came back, this time with Dolores, Dr. Hernandez greeted them with me, and we all settled into my office. I sat through the session unable to tell what they were talking about since everyone was speaking Spanish for the duration of the meeting. I was so relieved that they were able to talk in their own language and that Luis was free from the role of interpreter. The parents and Luis were all much more comfortable and animated. They had brought Luis's drawings back with them and brought some that Dolores had done on her birthday which showed her hugging her grandmother at the birthday dinner. I understood enough Spanish to gather that they were talking about Inez's death and how much she mattered to them. There were both tears and laughter during the session and I was profoundly grateful for Dr. Hernandez's willingness to see them with me.

After they left and Dr. Hernandez and I debriefed, he smiled and told me his guess had been right and that there was nothing to worry about with Luis, he was just fine. He shared with me that in some Mexican cultures, the living have regular communion with the dead and can invite deceased loved ones to visit with them. Because Luis and his grandmother had been so close, he still asked her to stay with him for a while as he went to sleep, a ritual that had been a part of his life from the beginning. Dolores had invited grandmother to her birthday party and Inez, of course, was there. In fact, everyone in the family reported visits with Inez following her death. All of the family members knew she had died, but her spirit was so strong in the family that she still visited when invited and each night they set a place for her at the table so Inez could join them if she liked. We called Luis's teacher and explained what had happened and she said she would invite Luis to share with the class some information about "Dia de los Muertes," (Day of the Dead) which was coming up in a few weeks to help them learn about his culture.

Lesson from the Big Chair: The Importance of Culture

How fortunate I was to have Dr. Hernandez work with Luis's family and me. I'm grateful that we weren't caught by the assumption that this was a manifestation of mental illness with Luis. I hate to think what might have happened for him if we didn't understand the cultural context. Luis was the black cat with the white stripe who fell in the stinky cheese and looked, walked, and smelled like a skunk, but wasn't. With Luis, I was an unconscious incompetent: I didn't know that I didn't know. Thanks to Dr. Hernandez, I moved up a level to conscious incompetent and started to learn more about Mexican culture. I keep a little retablo (figures of skeletons popular during "Dia de los Muertos" in Mexico) in my office to remind me to be curious and learn about other cultures before making conclusions.

PART II
HOW TO LOVE

The Buddha taught that the second challenge we face as humans is "How do I learn to love?" We are by nature interdependent; we need each other. Learning to build compassionate connections is vital to our survival and to the work of a psychotherapist. I'm delighted that I happened to choose a profession that has given me the opportunity to learn and practice compassion every day. The discipline of being in the big chair and opening my mind and my heart to such diverse and amazing individuals, my patients and students, has helped me learn the patience, hope, curiosity, humor, joy, sadness, and compassion that love encompasses. As I've heard patient's stories, shared their laughter and grief, I have come to love and appreciate people with deep reverence for each person's unique example of how to be human.

This profession also requires us to maintain a loving relationship with ourselves. I can't bring a compassionate presence to my work if I don't care about my own welfare and happiness. Buddha said that, "You yourself, as much as anybody in the entire universe, deserve your love and affection." We are tasked with doing what is necessary to build compassion toward ourselves and our experiences in order to be of help to others. Through learning to sit with our own suffering in a loving way, we build a mind that can bring compassion to the suffering of others.

Being a psychotherapist requires us to build emotionally intimate relationships with a wide variety of people. We work to become closely connected to others when they are at their worst: Angry, scared, hopeless, grieving, and alone. Learning to extend our capacity for compassion and connection is the focus of this section.

There are three chapters in this section that focus on different aspects of learning to love and build compassion. The chapters are:

- **Chapter 5: The Challenge of Compassion.** Those who work in this field are continuously challenged to learn how to extend compassion to those who may rarely experience it because of their behavior, illnesses, or conditions. Those who struggle with mental illness and/or addiction are often met with fear or contempt which produces a cycle of shame that feeds the illness. Isolation from human caring makes the sick sicker. Therapists are challenged to learn how to extend compassion toward those who are least likely to find it.

- **Chapter 6: Healing Through Connection:** The most important factor in the effectiveness of psychotherapy is the patient's sense that the therapist is genuinely concerned about them. Striving to make a compassionate connection to others can have a profound impact on therapists. Psychotherapy is often a very emotionally intimate experience for both patient and therapist. This chapter explores how therapists learn to connect to the sadness, fear, anger, hope, and joy that are shared in our work with patients.

- **Chapter 7: The Importance of Self Care:** The focus of this chapter is the on-going need for therapists to be aware of and take care of their own well-being. This is a lesson that is critical to having a career over time in the helping professions. Being a psychotherapist is tremendously hard work and learning to maintain a life apart from the work is a priority for longevity.

As the Dalai Lama notes, "Love is the wish to make someone else happy" (Kottler & Carlson, 2014, p. 53). That seems a good description of psychotherapy as well. When we learn compassion, which is love in action, we learn to heal both ourselves and others.

5

THE CHALLENGE OF COMPASSION

Learning Love

Learning compassion is one of the greatest gifts in psychotherapy, both for patients and therapists. Over time, this work can build a feeling of deep, heartfelt concern for other's well-being, regardless of who they are or what they have become. It doesn't happen with every client, but for those of us who stay in the profession, we often find that our capacity for compassion expands significantly. "By empathizing with someone who is more enraged, ecstatic, lonely, terrified, wildly loving, or terribly obsessive than you have known before, you gain the benefit of becoming familiar with a new emotional landscape, which will make it easier for you to empathize with others in the future" (Ladner, 2004, p. 128). Over decades of work in the big chair, I have experienced a profound expansion of compassion and empathy. As the illusion of "us" and "them" falls away, the distinction between what is good for me and what is good for you begins to merge. The desire to be of help to others becomes more integrated into who I am because we are all in the same boat. It's a simple concept that I will be healthier if you are healthier; I will be happier if you are happier; I will be safer if you are safer. "How can I help?" becomes a mantra and attitude that carries through our work and our lives. The compassionate perspective that we develop in the big chair can, hopefully, be more a part of who we are in all aspects of our lives.

I believe that compassion is an attitude that we can learn and, if we are truly to be of help to others, we must learn. In my study of Buddhist teachings, learning compassion has been a major focus. "Cultivating compassion is the single most effective way to make oneself psychologically healthy, happy, and joyful" (Ladner, 2004, p. xvii). A necklace that I wear every day has a depiction of Quan Yin, the Buddha of compassion. She attained enlightenment – freedom from earthly attachments and suffering – but refused to enter Nirvana, the Buddhist equivalent of heaven, until she could help everyone else go there with her. That's our compassionate nature, to want others to be free of suffering as much as we want that for ourselves. The desire to be happy and to avoid suffering is what connects us to each other and where the ability to be empathic begins. Even when there are no solutions to erase another person's pain, we can be a compassionate companion. We can bear witnesses to our shared human experience.

A Buddhist teacher gave me a lesson that was instrumental in helping me become more compassionate. He told me that I am the only person left on earth who has not attained enlightenment and that everyone else is still here in order to help me. It is my responsibility to learn from everyone I meet what it is I need to know. Sometimes it is patience, sometimes passion; sometimes perseverance, sometimes letting go; sometimes setting limits, sometimes inviting them in. My responsibility is to continually ask myself, "What am I learning from this encounter?" "How is this person being of help to me?" "What is this person trying to teach me that I need to know?" Everyone I meet has something to share that will help me, I just need to pay attention and try to understand what it is.

Love or Fear?

I believe that all our choices are between love and fear. Compassion is learning to make choices out of love instead of fear. As Gottlieb (2019) notes, "Therapy strives to teach you how to tell the two apart" (p. 234). That's a big challenge for most of us. We live in a culture that often encourages fear: Fear of the other, of losing out, of lacking something that we need, of being old, of loss, of death. Fear and the hatred and anger it can breed are endemic in our society. As I write this, for the past two years the U.S. has been pulling refugee children away from their parents and placing them in detention centers that are equivalent to prisons. This is a challenge to our compassion as a society. Our inability to make a compassionate response – to understand that if I would not want that to happen to my child, I don't want it to happen to your child – has been heartbreaking to me. Not only are we not in the same boat, but we are also treating those in the other boat as less than human. Learning compassion is critical not just for therapists, but for everyone if we want to live in a culture based on love instead of fear.

Compassion is a choice and an act of courage. We choose to reach out and join with those who are suffering from disorders that often frighten us. We choose not to look away from the problems and pain that addiction, mental illness, domestic violence, homelessness, and other social problems inflict on our neighbors. We commit ourselves to move toward, not away from, people when they are at their worst: Scared, hurt, angry, and in despair. We choose to acknowledge and even honor the humanity in everyone, regardless of who they are or what they've done. Choosing compassion as a career path is a way to make a life dedicated to learning love.

The Challenge of Stigma

Many of the people we work with are members of populations that are highly stigmatized and even demonized. Those suffering from addiction or severe mental illnesses are often ostracized and isolated. In movies and television, people suffering from psychosis are typically depicted as unpredictably dangerous (Tartakovsky, 2019). Heinous crimes such as mass murders are often blamed on "the mentally ill," which is simply untrue in all but a very few cases. According to data from MentalHealth.gov (https://www.mentalhealth.gov/basics/mental-health-myths-facts), "The vast majority of people with mental health problems are no more likely to be violent than anyone else. Most people with mental illness are not violent and only 3%-5% of violent acts can be attributed to individuals living with a serious mental illness." Fear, hatred, and anger are not mental illnesses. It's a double whammy that people with other types of disorders don't usually experience – being ill and shunned because of the illness. Sufferers must cope with both the disease and the stigma attached to it. If you tell someone you have cancer, they will probably offer sympathy and support: If you tell them you have bi-polar disorder, they will probably withdraw and avoid you.

Diseases associated with every other organ in the body generate loving responses, but brain diseases often generate fear. It's as though there's a contagious aspect to mental illness and a danger that if you try to connect, you'll be infected too. We seem able to envision ourselves having asthma or cancer, but not severe depression or schizophrenia. People with depression and anxiety disorders are expected to snap out of it, with addiction, they should just stop. We do not have those expectations for people suffering from diabetes or heart disease. For those entering the field, I urge you to be active as an advocate and educator in any way possible. We have an enormous task in helping the public better understand and care about the welfare of the mentally ill and addicted. I urge students to become active in supporting organizations like NAMI, The National Alliance on Mental Illness, (NAMI, 2019) which strives to provide accurate information about mental illness and addiction to the public and to educate policy makers and the media.

Not Everyone is Happy to Meet You

Being in close connection with people with mental illness and addictive disorders is challenging. It's usually the case that psychotherapists meet new patients when they are at their worst. People find their way to our offices when they are angry, frightened, overwhelmed, or feeling defeated. Seeking psychotherapy is usually the last choice when we are struggling with a problem, not the first. With addiction and severe mental disorders, people often come to treatment at the request of others or as a requirement of their employer or the courts. Not all people come to therapy as patients, some come through your door as combatants. I think it is an important experience to dedicate time in your career to working with people who are involuntary patients. Establishing a connection with someone who wants to avoid seeing you at all costs is a humbling and informative professional experience. For many involuntary patients, it is clear to them that I have nothing helpful to offer because "Nothing is wrong here" or "It's not my problem, it's my wife/court/boss that's got a problem." I've been described in creatively negative terms on many occasions. I've had to learn not to let someone's anger at the unfairness of being required to see me get in the way of my commitment to be of service to them.

I spent several decades working with court-ordered clients in substance abuse treatment programs and doing high conflict parental rights and responsibility assessments (commonly termed child custody evaluations). I've worked with hundreds of people over the years who viewed me as the enemy; someone they had to meet with in order to avoid certain consequences such as going to jail or not being able to reside with their children. Learning to establish and maintain a compassionate presence in this type of work teaches us a lot about patience and perseverance, both of which are important parts of a compassionate attitude. Supervision with senior clinicians who have spent significant time working with reluctant or hostile patients is invaluable. I have been so fortunate to have wonderful mentors and supervisors who helped me buckle my seatbelt in the big chair when learning to work with patients who wanted nothing to do with me. I also came to appreciate how important it is not to be isolated when doing this type of work. Having a support network of colleagues who appreciate the challenges is critical to serving these populations. When I worked in a group practice in Denver that focused on high conflict divorce and parental rights cases, we made a point of having lunch together to debrief and check in with each other. That really helped when I spent many hours a day with people who were often terribly upset with my decisions.

I had to learn to appreciate what creates the anger and avoidance that is at the core of challenging behavior for many involuntary patients. It is inevitably fear. That is understandable, there are threats and dangers to them in our relationship. I had to learn to build trust by addressing the fear directly and building an alliance with them to do our best to avoid the potential consequences. Regardless of my patient's attitudes, honesty, respect, and hopefulness on my part are required to open the relationship. Why would they trust me? I represent something that is threatening them. Acknowledging the patient's concerns and reluctance to see me as an ally is a critical step in making a connection. Regardless of what circumstance make it mandatory for them to meet with me, I strive to find a way to establish an empathic connection and build trust. I don't always succeed as the Case Study at the end of the chapter will illustrate.

The Paradox of Mental Illness and Addiction

The great paradox with addiction and some mental illnesses, such as schizophrenia, is that the person suffering is often the last to understand that they have a problem. For family and friends, the dilemma is that their loved one has become someone they don't know, someone they may have good reasons not to trust or to be afraid of in some way. It's enormously difficult to stay close to someone when they are in the throes of those illnesses. Seeing someone you care about not only struggling with addiction or a serious mental disorder but denying that anything is wrong is deeply painful and frustrating. It's easy to become irritated with them and angry that they can't see how they're hurting themselves and others.

I understand the challenge from my own experience with friends and family members who were changed beyond recognition when they experienced severe depression and anxiety or became dependent on alcohol or drugs. It's much easier to extend compassion to a patient that we only see for an hour or so a week, much harder when it's someone you are close to. In those relationships, I don't have the built-in barriers and protection of being in a professional role. I can't announce that "We're out of time for today" or make a referral to another helper. In therapy, we avoid the real risks that are inherent in people suffering from these disorders: The middle of the night call to bail them out of jail, the constant uncertainty of whether they are safe or not, the lies and threats, the nagging fear about what will happen to them and your relationship. When these dilemmas are affecting someone you love, there is anguish and fear that is very hard to mitigate, even for those of us who have spent a lifetime in the big chair. Ladner (2004) notes that "As we get to know others' minds, we learn to understand and work better with our own minds" (p. 128). It helps me appreciate the anxiety and constant worry that others feel when they are determined to stay connected to a loved one who is suffering so terribly. Remaining in compassionate connection to someone who doesn't realize the depth of their suffering and how it is affecting them is often a very hard choice.

If You're Afraid, Take Care of Yourself

Anyone who is ill suffers more if they are isolated from the care and comfort of others. As therapists, we are trained to step forward rather than back; to be first responders in the case of mental illness and problems such as domestic violence and child abuse. In these situations, there is always fear and often anger. You can expect that you will be treated badly by people who are scared and upset. I've sometimes requested that patients at least call me "Dr. Asshole." I also believe that we have a responsibility to be compassionate toward ourselves and respect that if we are in a situation that feels unsafe, exit as soon as possible. We should never be forced to work with a patient who threatens us or is unable to control aggressive behavior if we are working in a setting where we are vulnerable to attack.

My first job in the field in 1973 was as a ward attendant at a state hospital on a unit for people with chronic, severe mental illness. As I was going on the locked unit for the very first time, I held the door open as paramedics were taking another ward attendant out on a stretcher after a patient hit him in the head and knocked him out. I did momentarily consider going back to college and becoming a photographer instead. There are risks with this career, particularly in certain settings, such as prisons, or with some populations, such as domestic violence perpetrators. If your fear overcomes your compassion, take care of yourself first. There are times when it will be more important to extend compassion to yourself than to your patient. When you can't focus on the patient because your feelings are overwhelming, it's time to stop.

Motivational Interviewing

One of the most important lessons I learned is that we can be of help to others even when they don't want help. When books on motivational interviewing (Miller & Rollnick, 1991) and stages of change (Prochaska, DiClemente, & Norcross, 1992) first came on the scene, it was as though the heavens opened and the angels sang. Finally, there were guides to working with those who didn't voluntarily seek our help. There's an old joke that asks, "How many therapists does it take to change a light bulb? Just one, but the light bulb has to want to change." Now it's clear that we can work toward changing the light bulb regardless of whether it wants to change. In working with people suffering from addiction, waiting until they wanted to change was sometimes a death sentence. Motivational interviewing (MI) gave us guidelines to connect to those who needed help but were too disabled, fearful, or angry to seek it voluntarily. Understanding the stages of change let us learn how to target interventions to the patient's needs.

It is also a very respectful and compassionate approach that emphasizes empowering the patient to make choices. If you haven't already been introduced to MI, seek out the information and learn the approach, particularly if you are working with involuntary patients. I would not refer anyone to a facility for addiction treatment if the staff was not trained in using MI techniques.

The Limits of Compassion: Know When to Say No

Maintaining a compassionate mind while engaged in psychotherapy is largely dependent on self-awareness, particularly of countertransference and our own emotional triggers. Without an acute awareness of our reactions, biases, and assumptions, we aren't free to extend compassion to others. We can't be scared and compassionate simultaneously – it's an example of the need to make a choice between love and fear. Sometimes it important to be courageous, sometimes it's more important to honor your discomfort. To practice compassion, we must be willing and able to be present in someone else's suffering. When I talk about biases in my classes, I ask students to think about the issues or populations that they don't think they can work with. The students I have the most concern about are those who believe they can work with anyone, "no problem." I'll then share some experiences with patients who were perpetrators of horrible domestic violence, who abandoned their children because of substance abuse, who purposely tried to infect others with HIV when that was still a virtual death sentence, who were racist or sexist or hateful toward me and others. I want people new to this profession to understand how extraordinarily difficult it can be when you're in the big chair. If I couldn't find a way to manage my fear, I found other resources for them to get help. When I know I can't be present because of my fear, biases or beliefs, I also need to acknowledge that I can't be of help. "Compassion is only useful when coupled with clear-headedness" (Pipher, 2016). We need to know when to say "No."

Cozolino (2004) describes strategies to cope with patients who manifest frightening behaviors: First, don't panic; second, expect the unexpected, and third, don't try to reason with someone when they are irrational. Sometimes it's more important to be compassionate toward yourself and protect your own well-being.

"Clients with painful experiences and frightening symptoms are accustomed to living in a world where others avoid and reject them. Our ability to remain empathically connected to them through the expression of their suffering sets the stage for therapy to be a qualitatively different relationship experience – one where they are accepted, pain and all" (Cozolino, 2004, p. 42).

Everyone who works in this field will encounter patients with whom they struggle to maintain a compassionate presence. It's inevitable that those of us who have been in the big chair for many years have had occasion to "fire" a patient and have also been in a situation where we couldn't avoid working with someone although we wanted to escape. I've had times when the best strategy available was to alert other people in the office suite that I would be seeing a patient at 2:00 and to please call the police if they heard yelling or screaming. I sometimes warn aggressive patients that I have a weak stomach and am likely to violently vomit on anyone who tries to attack me. That seems to help, especially if I make a few retching noises when they become threatening toward me.

My first step when I believe I may be unable to work with someone is to seek supervision or consultation to see if there is something that I could learn or manage differently that would allow me to be of help to the patient. It's a delicate situation to inform a client that you aren't the right person to help them. There will be times when the most compassionate response we can offer is to help a patient find someone else. I am always clear I am making a referral because of my shortcomings, not theirs. It is my lack of understanding or experience that is the problem. Ethical guidelines require that we find alternative resources and refer the person to someone competent to help if we can't work effectively with them. I also make it clear that the referral is not because the person is "untreatable" or unworthy of help, instead they deserve to work with someone better able to be helpful to them.

Creating Compassionate Choices

Much of the work of therapy is to assist people in developing options for how they feel, think, and behave; an examination of how they evaluate their experience and make choices based on that assessment. The first law of cybernetics in physics is the "Law of Requisite Variety" which states that "The larger the variety of actions available to a control system, the larger the variety of perturbations it is able to compensate (Heylighen, 1992)." That translates to human behavior as predicting that the individual with the greatest flexibility of behavioral choices, when faced with a challenge, will have the most likelihood of finding a solution that works. The more choices you have, the more freedom you will feel, and the better quality of life you can have. For example, if I am employed at a clinic and I can do four different jobs in that organization, I'm more valuable to the organization than someone who can only do two jobs. The more options available to us and the more choices we can generate for how we'll respond to a situation, the better off we are.

I often say to patients, "You don't have to do the same thing again. The first time was a mistake, the second time is an opportunity to make a different choice." I might ask patients to assume the character of someone they know who truly cares about their welfare – a close friend or trusted family member – and talk to themselves from the perspective of that supportive person. If they're willing to do so, it helps them to build compassion for themselves as they learn to think from the perspective of a caring, trusted ally. With patients who had trauma early in their lives, such as sexual abuse or neglect, I might encourage them to talk to themselves as if they were the age when their trauma occurred and, as a loving adult, comfort that child within. The best way to learn compassion is to apply it to ourselves.

An important aim of psychotherapy is to help patients become more compassionate and accepting toward themselves. While you would rarely see it on their treatment plan, helping patients build a kinder, more caring relationship with themselves is the path to them being more satisfied in life, forming healthier relationships, and being better able to cope with all of the challenges that we face. "In therapy, we aim for self-compassion (Am I human?) versus self-esteem (a judgement: Am I good or bad?)" (Gottlieb, 2019, p. 120). I work from the belief that everyone does the best they can at any given time with the experiences, knowledge, and beliefs they have. We can only make choices according to what we have had the opportunity to learn. An important aspect of compassion is acceptance, not of what a person may be doing, but for the unique human being that they are. Rogers's (1961) concept of "unconditional positive regard," which is "the degree of positive affective attitude manifested by the counselor toward the client

(p. 47)," has consistently been shown to be a critical aspect of effective therapy (Bozarth, 2013). A therapeutic helping relationship is largely based on the clinician's ability to understand the patient's perspective and feelings from their point of view. The message to the patient is "I care about you" without the "if's" that are conditional. If I can extend compassion to them, they can learn to do so themselves.

Lessons from the Big Chair: Chapter 5

- Compassion is a state of mind that anyone can learn and develop.
- All our choices are between love and fear.
- Advocacy on behalf of the people we serve is an important aspect of our work and a way to increase both our own compassion and that of others.
- Maintaining a compassionate mind is reliant on self-awareness and an acknowledgment of our biases and fears.
- An unstated but significant goal of psychotherapy is to assist patients in developing more compassion for themselves as fallible human beings.

Case Study: Jacob

Jacob was a 35-year-old, white man who was assigned to me through the courts for monitoring of his interactions with his two children, boys age 7 and 10, and his ex-wife from whom he was recently divorced. I would be working as the Special Master with all the family members to help them enact the court's orders regarding the best interests of the children. I was trained in providing a shared parenting support program to high conflict, post-divorce parents with the goal of improving their communication as co-parents. When Jacob came into the office, his resentment and anger filled the room. Before I could get any information, he demanded to know if I was a "Christian" and "Did I believe in Jesus Christ as the highest authority regarding family matters?" I told him that I was raised in a Christian household and familiar with Jesus's teachings. I hoped that would satisfy him. It didn't. That wasn't good enough. I asked him what biblical teachings he felt were important regarding his circumstances in the hope that would help me better understand his concerns. His response was that "If you read the Bible, you would know." It was clear that he didn't regard me as anyone who could be of much help to him. I certainly couldn't compete with Jesus. Also, I was a woman, someone who, according to Jacob, had no authority over a man.

The judge's concerns were centered on Jacob's defiance of the court order that his ex-wife oversee their son's religious training. Jacob was involved with a cultish, extremely conservative church that only recognized the Bible as having any authority. Jacob was not compliant with most of the court's orders. He continued to take his sons to church meetings where they were prayed over and told that their mother was a sinner and doomed to hell for leaving their father. He persisted in contacting his ex-wife and harassing her about the "illegitimacy of the divorce." In a meeting with the boys, they described that they were told by their father to ignore their mother and do their best to reunite their parents. To Jacob, this is what God wanted from him, to convince his ex-wife that she needed to come back to him or lose her eternal soul.

The mother, Martha, had primary residential custody of the children and was increasingly concerned about what was happening with the boys. They were starting to do poorly in school, the younger boy was having nightmares about his mother being in hell, and both boys were increasingly angry and defiant. They blamed her for "destroying their family" and for and their father's distress. Martha shared that it was Jacob's affiliation with this church that ended the marriage. He had become verbally abusive, controlling, and impossible to reason with over the past few years and she finally couldn't abide what was happening for her and the children. He had alienated them from anyone who wasn't affiliated with the church. As the head of the family, he didn't tolerate any dissent from his decisions. The boys weren't allowed to play sports (which they both loved) or read anything that wasn't sanctioned by the church including some of their schoolbooks. Although Martha was also a Christian, she was alarmed at Jacob's behavior and concerned about the boys becoming increasingly isolated and anxious. For the sake of the children, she felt she had no alternative except divorce. She wanted the boys to have a relationship with their father and tried to work on a plan for Jacob to have the boys with him as often as possible. Any time she tried to talk with Jacob, however, she was confronted by his diatribe that she was sinful and a terrible mother for interfering with his authority as a father.

Jacob refused to come to any sessions with Martha unless she agreed to reconcile. That was not going to happen. This was quickly becoming an unmanageable case for shared parenting. I met with Martha separately given Jacob's inability to cooperate with the shared parenting structure of joint meetings. As a Special Master, I had the authority to make any recommendations to the court that I thought necessary regarding the parenting plan. It was clear that Jacob had no interest in my opinions or suggestions since I was not sufficiently versed in the Old Testament. During our meetings, he paced in the office and yelled at me that I had no authority and was damned for interfering in his family. I contacted his minister at the church who shared that he was also concerned about Jacob's behavior that was becoming increasingly hostile and aggressive. My concern was whether Jacob had an undiagnosed psychological disorder in addition to his religious fervor. His thinking certainly appeared delusional at times.

During our fourth meeting, Jacob became so loud and belligerent that I asked him to leave the office. When he refused, I left and went to a colleague's office to ask her to contact the police if she heard me yell "CALL." I returned to the office, opened the door, and again told him to leave, that the session was over. Fortunately, my files were locked in the cabinet and I had taken my notes with me. I could tell he had been looking for them. On the way out, he cursed me and said, "God will take care of you." His God was not known for compassion. I was shaking and afraid. I canceled the rest of my appointments for the day and spent some time with my colleague to calm down.

I decided to fire Jacob. Not only could I not do my job with him, but it was also interfering with my ability to be of help to my other patients. After meetings with him, I couldn't concentrate or calm myself enough to work with other patients. I wrote my resignation letter to the court as Special Master on the case with an explanation of my reasons and a recommendation that Jacob be reassigned to a male Christian therapist (if possible) and that he have only supervised visits with the children pending a complete psychological assessment. I contacted Jacob and canceled our upcoming appointments. I told him I would be contacting the court and what my recommendations were. He again cursed me and hung up.

I needed to protect my own well-being and knew that making a helping connection with Jacob was beyond my capabilities.

I saw Martha for a final session and shared with her my recommendations. She thanked me and said she would let me know how things were going for the children. I heard from her a few times, usually with concerns about Jacob's refusal to follow court orders. Jacob continued to pursue and harass her; he failed to comply with the psychological assessment order and refused to meet with any other therapist. He was limited to contact with the children at a visitation center where his interactions were supervised. Jacob continued, however, to contact the boys and coach them to convince their mother to come back to him. About four years later, I received a very unexpected call from Martha. She wanted to know if I could see her older son, now 14 years old. He was doing very poorly in school, frequently ran away from home (usually to Jacob's home) and had just been arrested for marijuana possession. I referred them to a colleague. I knew my limits.

Lesson from the Big Chair: Compassion for Myself

Like all relationships, therapeutic relationships end for different reasons. With Jacob, I was becoming increasingly afraid and angry, neither of which are conducive feelings for a therapy relationship. The fear I felt overcame my ability to be compassionate toward Jacob. I had to focus more on being compassionate toward myself. He was not a good patient for me, and I was not a good therapist for him. I enjoy challenging cases and have spent much of my career working with court-ordered and involuntary patients. Feeling threatened and unable to calm a situation with a patient is a red flag. Not only does the patient need to feel safe in our work together, so do I. I've rarely "fired" a patient but with Jacob, I made the right choice for both of us. I'm always reluctant to consider that, but there are times when we need to take care of ourselves instead of the patient. Admitting that you're in over your head is a good way to keep from drowning.

6

HEALING THROUGH CONNECTION

Compassion in Action

There's something about how we engage with other people that has a profound effect on our health and sense of satisfaction with life – we do best in connection to others (Pilgrim, Rogers, & Bentall, 2009). Research has consistently shown that a critical factor in the effectiveness of psychotherapy is the client's sense that the therapist genuinely cares about them (Duncan, Miller, Wampold & Hubble, 2010; Hoglend, Monsen, & Ronnestad, 2013). In Chapter 5, I explored the importance of developing a compassionate mind and attitude toward our work with others. In this chapter, I'll examine how we bring this into our relationship with patients. Demonstrating acceptance, compassion, and respect is intrinsic to helping others as a therapist. I agree with Kottler and Carlson (2014) that "…it is love that drives a lot of our therapeutic work" (p. 52). We usually avoid using that word when we talk about our professional work but in Buddhist philosophy, love is the wish to help others be happy. It's a love that is generated by a recognition of our shared humanity, equanimity, and connection to our shared experiences as human beings.

The therapist's most valuable resource is our sense of self and our ability to bring that to the therapy relationship. "We must demonstrate our willingness to enter into a deep intimacy with our patient, a process that requires us to be adept at mining the best source of reliable data about our patient – our own feelings" (Yalom, 2017, p. 40). We must commit to being open to bringing not just what we know but what we feel and our immediate sensations and reactions when we are in connection to our patients. The collaborative work of therapists and patients to transform or relieve suffering is central to our effectiveness. Psychotherapy is done with people, not to people. We learn to translate the love and care that we feel into actions that demonstrate deep compassion to our patients.

How we react to patients is usually a good indicator of how others experience them. The therapy office becomes a microcosm of the patient and therapist's worlds. Patients will not just tell us, they will show us what contributes to the problems they grapple with in life. Master therapists have learned to share with patients how we are impacted by their story and how it feels to be with them in the here-and-now. We must be aware of our reactions in order to give them honest, compassionate feedback about how we see them and how we feel about our encounter in therapy. For example, if a patient is going off on tangents or getting lost in the details of a narrative, I might respond that "I'm having trouble staying on the path with you because of the detours. Help me stay with what's important in your story so I don't get sidetracked. I don't want to get lost, so remind me of the purpose of what you're sharing." It may give me a sense of how others in their life may get lost or overwhelmed when they're speaking.

Being Present – Mindfulness in the Office

We let our patients know that we care about them by being fully present, listening attentively, and sharing our thoughts and feelings in the immediacy of our encounter. Fully present means that I commit to eliminating distractions; the phones and screens are put away (both mine and the patients) and the "In Session, Please Do Not Interrupt" sign goes on the door. More importantly, I spend a few moments before the session making an internal commitment to set aside distracting thoughts that might interrupt my concentration. I engage in a few moments of mindful breathing and focus on preparing myself to pay attention. Mindfulness practice creates a gap between my perception and my response which allows me to consider how to react and decide what to bring to the relationship at any given moment. Research (Aiken, 2006) has shown that psychotherapists who incorporate mindfulness practice into their work are more perceptive of their patient's inner experience and have a positive influence in cultivating empathy and building a more compassionate presence. Bishop et al. (2004) found that a more mindful state helps therapists become better able to connect to patients more dispassionately, without attachment, and to remain more reflective and less reactive. I have come to believe that creating a compassionate presence with patients is a critically important part of what I can offer.

After some discussion of mindfulness, if a patient is interested in doing so I begin sessions by sharing a brief mindfulness exercise with them. We devote a few minutes to focus on increasing our presence with each other. I will ask the patient if they would like to join me in preparing for our meeting by bringing our attention to the time we will spend together. To begin or session, I will use a mindfulness exercise like the following.

> Let us stop and become aware of our breath as we come together for our time today. We can gently close our eyes or let our focus soften as we sit comfortably, back straight but not rigid, feet on the floor, and hands resting on our lap. We'll follow our breathing for a few moments; breathing naturally, aware as we inhale of the air coming into our body and, as we exhale, of the breath leaving. As we become more aware of our breath and let our minds stay gently focused there, we commit to being fully present, to a full acceptance of the present moment, including how we feel and what we perceive. We give ourselves permission to let each moment be exactly as it is and allow ourselves to be exactly as we are. We breathe and let be. We move in the direction that our heart tells us to go with resolution and compassion for ourselves and others. After three more breaths, we'll open our eyes and begin our session.

I like sharing this practice with patients. It seems to create a break in the busyness of the day for both of us. It strengthens our commitment to the time together and helps us proceed with the intention to focus on compassionate interaction and contemplation. It's an invitation to be present with each other in a mindful way. It's never anything I would insist on as there are patients who might be uncomfortable with the practice for a number of reasons: It seems outside their religious or spiritual beliefs, they feel anxious about closing their eyes, being in their mind without distractions is highly stressful, and so forth. Even if the patient doesn't want to engage in this bit of mindfulness, I still silently bring myself to the session by slowing my breath and committing to the time I will be spending with the patient. I notice that even when we don't engage in the mindfulness exercise together, if I create a more relaxed, open presence, the patient often does too. There's a different energy in the room.

The Groucho Marx Dilemma

Groucho Marx (a comedian in the 1940's) once said, "I wouldn't want to belong to a club that would have me as a member." When we are at our worst and struggling with self-acceptance, it's hard to imagine that someone else could care about us. We've all been members of the Groucho Marx club at some point. It's a steep price for admission – a loss of self-respect, fear of intimacy, isolation, and, sometimes, self-destructive behaviors. When we don't want to be present in our own life, it's hard to imagine someone else would want to be around us. If I don't care about myself, only a fool would care about me. I think a lot of what is described as "resistance" is a fear of someone else seeing us as we see ourselves when we are in a dark place.

Finding the courage to invite someone to listen to our story is daunting when we feel more like the villain or victim than the hero of our narrative. We keep some things secret because we fear rejection and feel ashamed. We are already hearing the critic in our thoughts and don't want to face that same disapproval from anyone else. It still surprises me that we can do the work we do because it relies on people being willing to openly share the most painful, embarrassing, negative aspects of themselves. We invite those who seek our help to confront their hurt, fear, and anger through connection with us. We ask to be let into the places people hide, where they sit with their fears and hurt. It's an act of courage for both of us when we commit to the patient and therapist relationship and agree to visit those places where the pain lives.

What You Feel Matters

Practitioners new to the big chair often feel that they need to overlook or ignore their here-and-now reactions to patients during sessions and maintain a neutral façade. I believe that trying to create a blank slate of neutrality is a disservice to the process of psychotherapy. Being the "duck" (Chapter 4) doesn't mean you ignore your feelings and reactions. Psychotherapy is unique in that we focus on the here and now and provide immediate feedback to our patients about how we are impacted in our relationship with them. That is something we rarely have access to outside of the therapy office. Behaviors that are destructive or manipulative are usually met with fear, anger, or avoidance; when we are suffering from severe anxiety or depression, people may shy away out of ignorance about how to respond or because they feel overwhelmed. Rarely is there a compassionate, honest response from someone who is focused on our well-being.

Our willingness as therapists to share what we feel in the encounter with our patient is how we establish an empathic, healing connection. It's not a comment about what the patient is doing, it's about how you are affected by their behavior. Are you bored? Intimidated? Confused? Sad? Fearful? Compassionate self-disclosure of our reactions and feelings in a session is often what clients find most illuminating and useful. If I find myself feeling that I would rather be sitting in the dentist chair getting a tooth drilled than in my office with a patient, I need to pay attention to what is happening between us and stay present with that feeling. When a patient is wondering why they can't get further than a third date with someone, watch how they treat you during their third session and share your observations and reactions. The challenge then is to find a loving way to express my awareness to the patient so that he or she can hear it as useful information about how they are affecting me and possibly others.

No Matter Where You Go, There You Are

One aspect of being in the big chair that experienced clinicians are aware of is the almost constant sense of encountering our own dilemmas in our patients' narratives. It's eerie at times how patients' concerns reflect the exact issues that I am going through or surface unresolved issues in my life. We must be able to go where the patient goes, even when that leads us to a confrontation with our own shortcomings, faults, and heartbreaks. Being a psychotherapist requires us to become adept at establishing and maintaining a connection with others, but I inevitably find that it also entails an ongoing commitment to how I connect to my own life. If I'm working with a patient to help them relate more honestly with a spouse, I can't escape reflecting about my own relationship and how able I am to be open and truthful with my partner.

I find it especially challenging when a patient's struggles closely resemble my own. It's easy for me to get distracted, make assumptions, or jump to conclusions. I want to be exquisitely aware of feelings and projections that come up in those sessions and be conscious of how that is influencing or impacting our connection. I remember a young couple coming in to discuss their marriage plans and how to resolve some issues with the recently divorced parents of the groom who they worried might create problems at their wedding due to their ongoing anger and squabbling. The couple was so in love and excited about starting their life together as husband and wife. I met them as I was going through a painful, confusing, unexpected divorce when after a decade together, my husband had fallen in love with someone else. It was all I could do to not grab the young woman by the arms and tell her "RUN, JUST GO NOW!" I needed to be exquisitely careful that I didn't let my distress interfere with being happy for them and dedicating myself to helping them with their concerns. I remember them because working with them was actually helpful to me. It reminded me of how wonderful being in love was and the sensation of being excited and hopeful about the future. I hadn't felt that for a while, and it let me remember my former husband in a more kind and caring way. For many years, he had been a loving and devoted partner and we had enjoyed each other's company on many adventures. Although they never knew it, they assisted me in feeling grateful for what I had experienced in my marriage and in letting go of much of the pain I had been feeling. I did tell them how much I enjoyed working with them and that I would remember them with great fondness when we concluded our work together. That has certainly been the case.

We must care enough to tell our patients how it feels to be with them. We most effectively connect to patients when we compassionately share how we feel about our work together, not about what they are doing. I might tell a client that I'm very honored by their trust in disclosing something painful or secret or that their willingness to take a risk with me helps me feel more connected. "One just cannot see clients week after week, listen to their stories, and dry their tears without being profoundly affected by the experience" (Kottler, 2017, p. 10). It's both the blessing and curse of our profession that we are vulnerable to being emotionally impacted by our patients. It's what I love and fear the most about being in the big chair. Most of us have cried with our patients, laughed together, and shared in their anxiety about dangers present in their lives. I keep two boxes of tissues in the office, one for me and one for the patient. That deep connection to someone in pain is a transformative experience. Over time, it's made me much more tolerant of the mundane miseries of life such as bad drivers, long lines, and small aches and pains that I commonly encounter.

The Art of Confrontation

We establish trust by being courageous. Learning how to confront patients is a vital aspect of what we do in therapy. I describe confrontation as holding up a mirror, so the patient has a better idea of how their behavior is impacting both themselves and others. It is not the aggressive, self-serving type of encounter that is often our image of a social confrontation. Therapeutic confrontation is essentially helping the patient to engage in self-confrontation. The therapist is on the patient's side; it is done empathically with the goal of helping the patient face the impact, feelings, and reactions that their behavior is generating. The honesty and immediacy of an observation that a patient can get from a therapist is a rare opportunity to see themselves more clearly and take that information into consideration in determining their choices. There's no blaming or shaming, no "should" or "if you don't…," no anger or angst that accompanies the observation, just "Here's what I'm seeing or hearing," "How does that fit with what you want more or less of in your life?"

I look for the discrepancies between what a patient says they want and the behaviors that interfere with them meeting that goal. The purpose of confrontation is to empower the patient; to give them feedback that can assist them in making decisions about what to do. "There are often discrepancies in what clients say, and it can be deeply empathic to help the person articulate those discrepancies without judgment" (Martin, 2016, p. 55). I like to use a "Columbo" approach. Columbo was a television series about a seemingly bumbling detective who was a master at using his confusion as a way to confront crime suspects. He looked for the discrepancies: "You're saying you have insomnia and usually can't get to sleep until 3 a.m., but when your girlfriend called you at 10 p.m. and asked you to come over because she had gotten a threatening phone call from a neighbor, you said you were sound asleep. I'm confused about what happened there?" For me, it may be "You say you want to stop getting drunk but you're making plans to go out to the bar with your friends tomorrow night. How does that fit with your goal of sobriety?"

Most of us are understandably uncomfortable sharing a reaction that might sound negative. Confronting a patient with an observation that is challenging to them is risky. Confrontation that is therapeutic is a bit like stand-up comedy, it takes practice and a sense of timing. Avoiding it when needed, however, undermines our effectiveness and contributes to a lack of trust. Most of us know when we are behaving poorly and making choices that work against our best interests. To pretend with a patient that there's nothing problematic going on during our meetings with them undermines trust. If a patient has some sense that they are acting in ways that contribute to difficulties in their relationships and we don't acknowledge that in the therapy relationship, that sends the message that we're not willing to really engage and be honest. Confrontation is an important element of building trust; the assurance that we won't let our patient get away with behaviors that are harming them. We must be able to speak up when our patients are acting in ways that feel threatening or keep us in the dark about what's really happening. If we don't confront them, we are withholding critically important information that they are unlikely to get elsewhere.

Much of what I admire in my highly skilled colleagues is their ability to know what to share with a patient and, most importantly, how and when to offer a critical observation. Empathic confrontation is an art, one that takes a great deal of practice and a willingness to take risks. In our personal lives, sharing something with a loved one that you know may cause them distress is tremendously difficult for most of us. Those are situations that we prefer to avoid. Consequently, the art of compassionate confrontation is something that we must learn and practice if we are to be effective therapists.

Good supervisors are invaluable in helping us develop the skill of compassionate confrontation. I'm especially fond of either live supervision behind a mirror or reviewing videos of sessions when training new colleagues. We can begin to identify the "tells," those signs that the trainee is becoming disconnected or uncomfortable. I recognize my most common signals are looking repeatedly at the office clock, changing the subject, and spending more time talking in the session than the patient does. When I engage in those, I know it's time to pay attention to what I'm feeling in the session. There are clues that supervisors can see that may be out of our awareness. If you haven't already, find a supervisor who can spend time helping you learn your signals. Being able to recognize, acknowledge, and process that information with a patient is likely to be valuable.

Finding the Pony

One of the most important things that we can offer our patients is hope. Hope is what empowers us to take risks and change course. During a crisis, we all struggle to imagine a life we can find satisfying and meaningful. When you're afraid you are drowning it's hard to recall sitting safely on the shore. Entering psychotherapy is often the last resort for people; they have already tried other solutions that didn't help. "Because people are coming to therapy for their problems, it is easy for both client and therapist to get tunnel vision and forget to see the positive aspects of their lives" (Cozolino, 2004, p. 53). One of the most important things a therapist needs to learn is often overlooked in clinical training programs: How to look for the pony. I share the following story with my students.

> Some behavioral researchers were interested in finding out how children cope with highly negative environments and designed the following study. There was a door with an observation window leading into a large room where the researchers could observe their subjects. Two subjects were selected, both 11-year-old girls who were of the same height. They were told that they were going to be placed in the room one at a time and observed, but that they could leave any time by knocking on the door. The first little girl is led to the door, the door opens, and she is pushed into the room. To create a negative environment, the room was filled with horse shit up to chin height for the girls. After just a few seconds in the room, the first girl is screaming to be let out and pounding on the door. The researchers let her out and ask her about her

experience. "It was HORRIBLE, I can't believe you did that to me!" She's crying and very upset. They calm the girl down, gather their data, make their notations, and send the first girl away. They then bring the second girl to the door. The door is opened, and she is pushed into the room filled with horse shit. Through the window, they see her beginning to move slowly around the room, but soon, she begins to laugh and starts flinging horse shit in the air as she moves everywhere in the space. After 20 minutes, she's still laughing and flinging horse shit and they decide to invite her out. She reluctantly comes to the door, covered in horse shit but smiling and still giggling. They ask her about her experience, and she tells them simply, "I was looking for the pony."

It's a therapist's job to look for the pony, even when it appears that it's just a room full of shit. I believe that one of the most overlooked aspects of clinical training is that we are not very well prepared to recognize and assess the positive, effective, healthy behaviors and beliefs of our patients. If we don't recognize what those are in our patients, we certainly can't help them be more aware of their strengths. I often determine whether a counseling skills textbook will be adopted for my courses based on the subject index. Is there compassion, confrontation, and hope in that index? Those are vital attitudes and skills to learn in order to become an effective psychotherapist.

Employing a more positive vocabulary is an important part of introducing hope and building confidence. Therapists have established an enormous, nuanced, detailed dictionary to describe pathology and problems. We need the equivalent of a Diagnostic and Statistical Manual of Mental Disorders (American Psychiatric Association, 2013) that focuses on assessing the positive aspects of who we are. Is our patient creative? Resilient? Persevering? Do they have a good sense of humor? Can they tolerate discomfort and uncertainty? Are they compassionate and connected to others? Do they assume responsibility for their behaviors and choices? Are they kind? Generous? We need to have the ability to get in the room full of shit with them and search for the pony. Establishing hope relies on our ability to hold a mirror up to patients that lets them see what helpful experiences, traits, and beliefs they bring to psychotherapy. In addition to confronting the discrepancies, I want to confront them with their strengths and examples of good choices they've made. We both acknowledge the shit in the room but believe firmly that there's a pony in there somewhere. That's my foundation for finding hope.

So, how do we find the pony? First, we must have an unshakeable belief that there's one there. Regardless of how messy and problematic a patient's life has become, the reason they are with me is to clean up that mess. We learn to look past the chaos to find order. It helps to appreciate that chaos, and the crises that spin out of it, actually set the stage for new order and stability to emerge (Butz, Chamberlain & McCown, 1997). When we simply can't keep doing what we've been doing, it's time for a change. As the Asian symbols for the word crisis indicate, crisis is a combination of danger and opportunity. If we get caught in the illusion that there's nothing useful in a patient's life, that it's just a room full of shit, then we will also run crying from the room at some point. Believe in the pony, it's there somewhere.

The first step in finding the pony requires being intently focused on listening for information about the patient's life, both past and present, which has a positive, healthy aspect. Are they resourceful? Engaging? Funny? Thoughtful? Some questions to elicit this information are, "What would someone who knows you well tell me that they like most about you," "What is an aspect of yourself that you would never want to give up?" "What are some things that you regularly do that make you happy?" I want them to give me a description of the pony from their perspective. It's important for me not to get locked into a description of their best self that doesn't fit with what they believe. Most of us endure some level of annoyance when someone attempts to compliment us in a way that simply doesn't fit our self-perception. The pony can't be phony, it must resonate with how the patient sees themselves. Effective therapists know how to work with what they've got, not with what they might want.

Finding the Positive with Reluctant Patients

I believe that even with involuntary patients, those who are with us because someone else thinks they need help, we must search for the pony. People are always free to ignore a court order or ultimatum from a boss or partner. Certainly, there will be consequences for that choice, but many take that path rather than getting involved in therapy. With those patients who do choose to see me, regardless of how reluctantly, I invite them to join me on the search for the pony. I ask them, "What is something you're proud of that you want me to know about," "Tell me about a bad decision you made and how you overcame that?" or "Think of a problem that you have successfully resolved." I've yet to meet anyone who doesn't have some experience of feeling competent or proud of an accomplishment in their life. Look for ponies both large and small: They learned to speak a second language, they left an abusive relationship, they helped their son learn to ride a bike, they figured out how to stay alive on the streets during the winter. Everyone has something they like about themselves that they wish other people could see in them. I want to know what that is and make it an important part of building our connection.

I encourage reluctant patients to share things that they feel good about in their life, what they like about themselves, what they wish others knew that would help them feel more understood. Particularly with patients who might be hesitant or even hostile to being in therapy, connecting with positive aspects of themselves can help to reduce the fear that I'm just another "expert" who is going to blame or label them. Even if they can't or won't engage with that exploration, I point out that "It takes a lot of courage to even come to meet with me. I know you didn't have to; you could have instead taken whatever consequences came your way. I appreciate that you're here." I also want to be clear that I'm on their side and I'm working for their welfare regardless of whether someone else made them seek help. I'm very clear about what I may be required to disclose to others (e.g., the court or their employer) but that my main purpose is to help them in any way I can. I assure them that they will have access to any reports or information about them that I'm sharing with others and secure a release of information even when it's already clear that the judge or their boss has access to my findings. Establishing trust with reluctant or involuntary patients is critical for any meaningful work is to occur.

I also want to know about any time in their life that they felt safe, competent, understood, happy, or satisfied. Have they found the pony before in their life? I might encourage them to "Tell me about a time in your life that you felt safe or happy." "If you could go back to any single experience in your life, what would it be?" "What about that time was most important for you?" I particularly focus on how they contributed to those positive experiences and what they did to make those times happen. Most likely, they haven't always been in a room full of shit. At some points, they were able to enjoy a ride on the pony.

Finally, I build with them a sense of hope that they can clean up the mess. I've learned to be clear in my thinking that I am not the one responsible for fixing someone else's life. If we approach patients as people who need to be "fixed" that means we will treat them as if they are broken. We are a character in their life story, but they are the author. Often, you will see hope for a patient before they do. As you get a better picture of the pony, share it with them with conviction and enthusiasm. Most of us have had the wonderful gift of someone who believes in us, who sees the potential and the good in us. I sometimes lament that there aren't cheerleaders for those of us who got through a betrayal without becoming bitter and vindictive, who experienced profound losses but didn't fall into despair, who reached out to help others even when we were suffering. Those things are truly worth cheering about so keep some pom-poms in your office and use them.

NOTES FROM THE BIG CHAIR

We use the power of our presence to build connection. "A therapist who is vibrant, inspirational, and charismatic; who is sincere, loving, and nurturing; and who is wise, confident, and self-disciplined will often have an impact through the sheer force and power of her essence..." (Kottler, 2017, p. 3). Your theoretical orientation and the specific techniques that you've learned aren't the important factors in making an effective connection to a patient: You are. You can't fake this stuff. Empathic confrontation, empowering patients, and bringing hope to our work are important skills, but more importantly, they're reflections of who we are. We are people who engage in the hard work of loving those who may feel unlovable. We are brave companions to others who are in horrible pain and despair. Our healing presence is a mixture of compassion, curiosity, confrontation, courage, and hope. That's what a therapist's pony looks like. Saddle up and ride in.

Lessons from the Big Chair: Chapter 6

- Connection is based on trust and hope.
- My job is to be present and aware of myself in the relationship – how I'm being affected, how it feels for me to be with a patient, and what

I might be bringing to the relationship that will help or hinder their progress.

- It takes courage to be connected to people who are suffering and to confront the ways in which they create aspects of that suffering.
- We must be willing to acknowledge and share our perceptions and reactions for the benefit of the patient.
- As a therapist, we must have an unshakable belief that there's a pony in the messiness and chaos of our patients' lives and be able to dig in and help them find it.

Case Study: Theresa

Theresa was referred to me by her physician following a car accident in which she was seriously injured. Following the accident, she developed panic attacks and a degree of anxiety that made her unable to drive and it was difficult for her to even be a passenger in a car. Because the physician knew I practiced EMDR (Eye Movement Desensitization and Reconstruction) (Shapiro, 2018), she referred the patient for help managing her anxiety. EMDR therapy is an interactive psychotherapy technique used to relieve psychological stress based on trauma. I had trained with its founder, Francine Shapiro, and used it successfully with many patients who were suffering from Post-Traumatic Stress Disorder (PTSD).

When I went to meet her, Theresa was seated in the corner of the waiting room, hidden behind a large magazine she was reading. When I approached her and spoke her name, she was clearly very uncomfortable. As I shook hands and introduced myself, I could feel her hand trembling and was aware that she looked at the floor as I led her to the office. She was a single, white woman in her early 30s, moderately overweight, with curly blond hair. In the office, she again sat in the corner of the couch, as far away from me as possible. Her anxiety was like a force field that surrounded her. I worried I might scare her away like a deer that gets startled if I come to close.

During the initial interview, she spoke in a quiet voice and rarely looked up from the floor. I always invite new patients to ask me any questions they might have before starting the interview. She had never seen a therapist before but had no questions for me. Theresa shared that she was coming to see me only because her physician had asked her to and that she didn't think I could be of much help. I assured her that our first meeting would help us both determine if working together might be useful for her. Theresa reluctantly described the car accident and the anxiety that had invaded her following that event, making it almost impossible for her to function. Theresa was missing work, isolated, and fearful she would lose her apartment if she lost her job. Driving was a nightmare for her. She clearly had Post Traumatic Stress Disorder (PTSD) symptoms: Nightmares, situational triggers that made her feel unsafe (such as driving or being in a car on busy streets), flashbacks to the accident, and difficulty in sleeping and eating. In the accident, her pelvis had been crushed and she required both surgery and physical therapy for many months before she was able to return to her apartment where she lived alone. She had stayed with a sister during her recovery.

When I asked about her family, she again became very anxious and I noticed her hands shaking again. She was the youngest child with an older brother, Jim, and older sister, Arlene. She related only basic information about her family and declined to answer some questions. She did admit that there were addiction problems with her brother and possibly with an uncle on her mother's side of the family. Along with talking about the accident, sharing information about her family also created a great deal of discomfort for her. I tucked those observations away to return to later if she stayed with me in therapy.

Her main concern and the reason for the referral was to reduce the anxiety so that she could resume functioning independently. We reviewed the procedures for EMDR, I gave her some information to read to help her determine if she wanted to try the process if she chose to return. By the end of the interview, Theresa was comfortable enough to say she would come back again, and we set up an appointment for the following week. At the second session, she committed to trying EMDR and we began that process. In the screening, she stated she didn't have any other history of trauma other than the accident. She was a good candidate and responded well to the initial trial using the technique. Theresa stayed with the process during that session and was able to get some reduction in her overall anxiety about the accident. She decided she wanted to continue our work and during the next few EMDR sessions, she was able to recall images of the accident without severe anxiety and reported fewer nightmares and enough comfort to drive herself to work and to shop for groceries.

During what was to be our final session of EMDR, we were working on reducing the body discomfort that she had experienced in her pelvic region since she carried a lot of her physical tension there and still had residual pain from the accident. That session provoked a very strong response as I asked her to focus on the physical sensations in her pelvis, abdomen, and groin. She started shaking and sobbing uncontrollably. We stopped the EMDR and I asked her what had come up for her. Theresa shared that she had been sexually assaulted as a child at about age 10 but hadn't recalled any memories or thoughts about that for a very long time. That confession certainly helped me understand her initial fear about seeking therapy. She must have worried that at some point we might uncover her hidden history.

Rather than opening that issue further, I helped her to calm down and we set another meeting with the understanding that she could share more about that if she wanted to in the next session. I reminded her to write down anything she wished to talk about with me in her journal. At our next session, she was very reserved and quiet again, avoided eye contact and was clearly anxious, much as she had been at our first meeting. In a way, it was a first meeting with the Theresa who had been harmed as a child. All the trust we had built together through the EMDR sessions would need to be rebuilt and be much stronger if she was to tolerate opening the secrets about her abuse. It's often the case that current anxiety and pain (for Theresa, the car accident) link us to times when we had those feelings previously.

That was certainly true for Theresa. She had been depressed for much of the prior week and had some trouble with nightmares again, but the current dreams were about the sexual abuse. She was a very modest, shy woman, and didn't want to go into any detail. I wanted to establish that both she and others were not in any danger from her attacker, so asked if she could disclose who it was. Theresa said it was an uncle, her mother's brother Luke, who had visited her family and that it had only occurred on one occasion. She claimed that the uncle had been deceased for over 20 years; he died in a car accident while he was intoxicated.

Theresa was very reluctant to talk about any details of what happened. My approach is to be very respectful and patient when beginning to talk about trauma history so long as there is no immediate or ongoing threat.

I appreciate how painful this type of work can be. She never told anyone about the sexual assault but did tell her mother after the incident that "I don't like Uncle Luke" and he was never invited back to their home. She said that she remembered her mother becoming angry when she told her she didn't like him, but she wasn't angry with her, she was angry with Luke. I wondered if Theresa's mother had also been victimized by her brother when she was young. Fortunately, Uncle Luke didn't visit the family again. Theresa remembered when she heard that he had died. Her family didn't go to the funeral and she remembered her mother saying, "Good riddance."

Theresa and I continued working together for the next 3 years. She was one of my longest-term patients. We worked together on processing the sexual abuse and how that had affected her development, particularly her social life. She had never dated and avoided any intimate contact. She felt ashamed of what had happened but was able to appreciate that she was a child who wasn't able to protect herself when the abuse occurred. Theresa had, however, protected her mother, who had bouts of depression and anxiety, by not telling her about the molestation. During our work together, Theresa became more involved in social activities through her church and met a man named Jim who asked her out. When Theresa told me this, she broke down in tears and couldn't speak for some time. I handed her tissues and waited until she could catch her breath. "What happened Theresa? It's clear that there's something very upsetting about meeting Jim." She was again shaking, something that I hadn't seen for almost 2 years. "Jim is my brother's name" she said as she stared at the floor. I asked, "Can you tell me what's happening. Do you feel safe sharing with me what brought up these tears?"

Her first response was, "I'm sorry, I hope you won't be angry with me." I assured her that I wouldn't be upset with her regardless of what she shared. Theresa finally had the courage to tell me that "I wasn't molested just by my uncle, it was also my brother, Jim." Her older brother, Jim, had begun sneaking into her bedroom when she was five and his abuse continued until she was 12 and started having her menstrual periods. He kept her quiet by telling her that their parents wouldn't believe her and that he'd kill her and her sister if she told. Jim had a rifle that he threatened her with many times. For most of her childhood, she feared for her life as she struggled to keep a horribly painful secret.

After almost three years, she finally was able to tell me about his sadistic abuse and her childhood filled with fear. As an adolescent and adult, Jim was addicted to alcohol and drugs and ran away from home shortly after he stopped abusing her. She had no contact with him after he left and found out that he had died almost 10 years ago while in prison. When her new friend, Jim, asked her out and kissed her at the end of their first date, she found herself overwhelmed by guilt and fear. We continued together in therapy for another year to work through her childhood trauma and help her make a healthy adjustment to the new aspects of her life including her first romantic relationship with James. She asked Jim if she could call him James instead and was able to share some of her backgrounds with him over that year. When we finally ended our work together, she and James were living together, Theresa was back at work, and she was planning her wedding.

Lesson from the Big Chair: Patience

I was so grateful that Theresa had the courage and determination to stay with me in psychotherapy for the four years that it took for us to sort through all that she brought to that endeavor. Although she came in at the request of someone else, finding some relief from her immediate anxiety helped her be more willing to engage with psychotherapy. It was an important lesson to me in patience and letting the story unfold in its own time. When someone has a long history of traumatic abuse, trusting others is a terrifying leap of faith. It was an honor that she let me be the one to hear her story and that she was also willing to be patient with me. I'm so grateful that we both were able to stay connected long enough for Theresa to finally tell her true story.

7

THE IMPORTANCE
OF SELF CARE

Taking Care of Yourself is a Requirement

I would be suspicious of any book about life as a psychotherapist that didn't devote attention to our need to take care of ourselves. Self-care is not an option, it's a requirement. All professional ethical standards emphasize the importance of doing what is necessary for us to function effectively in this role. When we are struggling, we need to seek consultation and therapy for ourselves. Because much of what brings people to this profession is a compassionate desire to be of help to others, our training and ethics need to remind us that self-care and an on-going commitment to our own well-being can't be ignored. Research has demonstrated that even if we aren't aware of the impact, patient ratings of the quality of their alliance with their therapist are lower when they are aware that their therapist is experiencing personal distress (Nissen-Lie, Havik, Hoglend, Monsen, & Ronnestad, 2013). We are obligated professionally to protect our patients from the negative impact our own emotional or physical problems might create in the therapeutic relationship. More importantly, we can't give what we don't have. If we want to be a compassionate presence in the lives of others, we must also apply it to ourselves.

Therapy is hard work emotionally, cognitively, and physically for us as well as our patients. Being fully present in sessions takes a great deal of energy. There's a lot more to what we do than just sitting comfortably and listening to someone talk. Clinicians in training or early in their careers often get a clear sense of how exhausting a day at the office or clinic can be. Duncan (2014) accurately notes that "We have to put ourselves out there with each and every person, each and every interaction, and each and every session. It is a daunting task, to be sure, but one that is perpetually minimized in its importance and difficulty" (p. 166). Our emotional state will inevitably impact our ability to be present in our work. We must strive to meet the same standards for self-care and well-being that we encourage in our patients.

One of the most asked questions from students in training is "How do you keep from taking everything home with you?" What they really want to know is how do you turn off the therapist role and have a life of your own. It's an important question. As noted, psychotherapy is hard work. Those of us who have stayed in the profession over several decades have done so because we learned (sometimes the hard way) to take care of ourselves. We ignore self-care at our peril. I have had students during their first semester of internships decide that this profession is not for them. The amount of emotional energy and the challenge of being connected to people in profound distress can be overwhelming. The demands can easily become more of a task then we are prepared to accept. In this profession, there is always more to do than there is time to do it. "If we don't care for ourselves we can become as depressed, anxious, or angry as our clients" (Pipher, 2016, p. 76). You can't help someone else find the light if you're stumbling around in the darkness.

Psychotherapists are Human Beings

Everyone experiences loss, physical decline, illness, heartbreak, uncertainty and all the other dilemmas that come with being human. For therapists, there is a danger of becoming captured by the illusion of "having it all together" when it comes to coping with our own problems. We learn to keep our experiences out of the conversation with clients, except in those instances when it can serve a therapeutic purpose for them. Sometimes, therapy is a very lonely profession because we become good at keeping our own needs and concerns out of the dialogue. It can be difficult to be spontaneous as we consider what impact our comments or self-disclosure might have on a patient. I sometimes experience reluctance to enter conversations in social situations because I've become used to monitoring myself and listening rather than speaking. I also find that having highly intimate, meaningful interactions with patients can make social "chit chat" seems frivolous or uninteresting. We become very good at editing ourselves and thinking about how to best share personal information in our work and that can impact our social and intimate relationships. I spend a lot of time during a workweek NOT talking about politics or celebrities or what's on television. The longer I've been a therapist, the worse I've become at small talk.

The paradox of being in the big chair is that while we are guarding against inappropriate self-disclosure, we are also taught to be acutely aware of our inner world and reactions to what clients are sharing with us. The importance of countertransference is ingrained in us through our training. So, there we sit, highly aware of our reactions and how a patient's story is affecting us yet cautious about expressing feelings or thoughts based on our experience. This can leave us with an accumulation of strong emotions and memories that we must hold and find a way to work through.

The Therapist in Therapy

Throughout my career, there have been times when I realize that I need to talk about something I'm going through. It may be something personal or professional that is troubling me. My first clue that I'm feeling that need to talk is a longing for someone to ask, "How are *you* doing?" We so often assume that our physicians are healthy, that our dentists don't have a toothache, and that therapists don't have life problems. Patients and students often believe we have a perfect, wonderful life with conflict-free relationships, well-adjusted children, financial security, and all the other trappings of a fully realized, happy existence. Because of the need to limit self-disclosure in our work, we inadvertently contribute to that fantasy. Our training to appear calm and our attention to effective communication skills and relationship building create an illusion of invulnerability to the challenges that everyone experiences. Don't fall for that yourself. Be human. Ask for help. Take time to sit on the couch and find someone to listen to you.

Especially for those of us in private practice, it can become easy to be isolated and find ourselves wrestling alone with strong feelings from our work. That's one reason why it's important to seek help for ourselves. In order to protect confidentiality, we can't go to friends and family to talk about experiences in the big chair, particularly if it is something triggered by a session with a patient. One of the dilemmas of being a therapist over many years is that you get very good at listening. It can become a dilemma because others come to expect that from you. It's not unusual for me to have a conversation with a friend and realize, as we're ending our time together, that I haven't said anything about how I'm doing. Sometimes, I'm not asked and sometimes I duck the question as I'm accustomed to doing at the office with "I'm good, thanks. Now, how are you?" A study of therapists who engaged in therapy found that over 90% felt it was very helpful (Bike, Norcross, & Schatz, 2009). "One of the great values of obtaining intensive personal therapy is to experience for oneself the great value of positive support" (Yalom, 2017, p. 13). In a conversation with my colleague, Erika Remsberg, we shared what a relief it is when we see a therapist for ourselves. Finally, someone who really listens to us and lets us talk at length about our lives.

I periodically need to give myself what I strive to give my patients; someone who is there for me. I live in a small, semi-rural town in Florida, and finding a therapist that I don't have some type of personal or professional acquaintance with is daunting. I've found it's better to travel further and find a therapist who is outside my area. I look for someone who is appropriately credentialed, not bound to any particular theoretical orientation or techniques, and, most importantly, a person with whom I feel comfortable and safe. Warmth, respect, kindness, attentiveness, and competence are what counts for me, just as I believe it does for the patients that I see. I also look for little "tells," things that give me some sense of who they are. What's on their bookshelf? Do they start and end sessions on time? Is their office comfortable and uncluttered (I especially notice if they have papers or files out where I can see the names of other clients)? Do they put away their phones and screens when we meet? I once had a supervisor caution me to never see a therapist with dead plants in their office. I pay attention to the small details that indicate this therapist is paying attention to how their environment reflects who they are. Most importantly, being in therapy myself more finely tunes my empathic appreciation for the anxiety that patients often bring; will I be understood and accepted? I trust that being a patient will help you appreciate more deeply how comforting it is to have a concerned, supportive therapist in your life.

"Psychotherapist" is a Hard Role to Step Out of

Another dilemma that Yalom (2017) so accurately describes is that "… patients are so grateful, so adoring, so idealizing, we therapists run the risk of becoming less appreciative of family members and friends, who fail to recognize our omniscience and excellence in all things" (p. 252). As I'm preparing to retire and cut back on the hours that I spend teaching and at my practice, I'm acutely aware that I'm going to miss the respect and deference that is often afforded to me. I like being perceived as the kindly, wise old woman. I even have a t-shirt that says, "Never underestimate an old woman with a psychology degree." There is a great deal of gratification that I've had from occupying the big chair. I'm grateful that psychotherapy is a profession that rewards the wisdom that we accumulate as we mature. Unlike many other professions, we can age gracefully as a psychotherapist.

Being adept at helping others isn't always a welcome role for those with whom we have family or social relationships. When you've spent decades honing your awareness of problematic patterns in relationships and clues that someone is struggling with an emotion or experience that's hurting them, you can't just not see things. Also, I'm used to people listening to me and even taking notes at times. With friends and family, I struggle to be heard just like everyone else. I find it difficult not to step in and offer feedback or share my observations. It's painful for me if I want to talk over something that's happening in an intimate relationship with a friend or partner and am accused of "acting like a therapist." I'm sure plumbers can ask a partner "How are you feeling about what just happened?" and not be perceived as having ulterior motives. It feels unfair at times. I have learned to lead with my own thoughts and feelings instead of asking about my partners'. It's that shift of putting myself in the foreground with my personal relationships that I studiously avoid in the therapy relationship. I frequently need to remind myself that I'm not in a helper role and step back and focus on my needs and how to best express them.

The Demands

One aspect of this profession is that there are always demands that we must learn to manage. I encourage those beginning their career to build self-care into their schedule. Set your limits and stick to them. There was a brief period in my private practice when I was seeing 10 patients a day, 5 days a week. After a few months, I found that my ability to concentrate was impaired and that I was taking files home with me and working several hours a night after my full days at the office. The effect of my behavior became evident when I fell asleep in a session with a patient. She was the fifth session of the day and I had not taken a lunch break in order to fit in more appointments. I dozed for about 10 minutes and awoke to find a very unhappy patient staring at me. Despite my apology, she rightly decided not to return the following week and didn't respond to my attempts to reschedule or refer. Following that, I changed my schedule to include a break for lunch and a short walk and I saw fewer patients. After 30 years, however, I still feel bad about that incident and hope that she found someone else to talk with. If you are exhausted and overwhelmed, you will communicate that to patients. Learn to say "no" and to ask for help when you need it. There is always more work than you can possibly do.

Get a Life

The colleagues that I worry most about are those who seem to have little going on in their lives aside from their work. They are always "on," when they're socializing it's with other therapists, they don't go on vacation or limit the hours of their practice. This is a profession that will take as much room in your life as you allow. The work is never done, someone always needs something from you, there are always articles to read and paperwork to do. If you are someone who needs to have everything done before you relax, prepare to be stressed on a permanent basis. Setting limits and stepping away when it's time to go are vital to preventing burn out and exhaustion.

In his book "The Making of a Therapist", Louis Cozolino provides useful guidelines for keeping your own sanity as you build your career. I believe his points are worth exploring. He suggests:

- Know your limits and select your clients.
- Keep perspective.

- Watch out for traumatic contagion.
- Know your laws and ethics.
- Engage in consistent self-care (Cozolino, 2004, p. 188–195).

Know Your Limits

If you know that there are certain populations or issues that you aren't prepared to work with or which would be highly stressful given your values, beliefs, or biases, honor your limits. You will be of no help to someone you don't feel safe around or don't believe you can help. I know that I do not work effectively with patients with eating disorders or compulsive hoarding, despite having some training and supervision with these issues. I just find those disorders baffling and difficult to understand. I also don't work with child predators. As a member of Bikers Against Child Abuse (BACA), I am devoted to empowering abused children. I can't work with a child abuser and not think about the boys and girls I know who struggle daily just to be a child again and not be afraid of the world in which they live. I'm grateful for dedicated colleagues who can work with the people that I can't. I know that people who abuse children often have a history of being abused and certainly need and deserve competent care. I'm just not a good match for working with that population. If I use my time and resources to try and help someone I feel very uncomfortable with or incompetent to assist, I have less energy to give to my other patients. I keep referral information handy so that I can help those I can't help to find someone who can.

Keeping Perspective

Keeping perspective means developing ways to let the work stay at the office. It helps to realize that we are engaged in helping people when they are at their worst. I am willing to accept that I will fail to help some people; they're not ready, I'm not ready, the relationship doesn't work out, things get in the way, I get in the way. This is a treacherous profession for those who see themselves as the Lone Ranger or a superhero who can swoop in and right the wrongs of someone else's life. I tend to let myself be seduced into working with challenging cases, particularly those who have seen other therapists with limited success. I'm getting better after 40+ years of saying "No, but thanks for thinking of me" when I get those referrals if I really don't have the resources or time to take one. If I do accept the challenge and find myself joining the patients' list of impotent or bungling therapists, I find it helpful to just accept that patients have a right to hold on to problems that they aren't ready to let go of. I can only do what I can do. People come to therapy with complicated concerns and needs. We have a role to play but it isn't to save everyone from their lives. When it's time to stop work for the day, go home, play with your kids or pets, have a nice meal, take a walk, read a juicy novel or just do something else.

Watch for Traumatic Contagion

Traumatic contagion is endemic in our field. Being closely connected to people who have been through trauma is itself traumatic, particularly if it triggers something in your own experience. It is painful for me to delve into a patient's trauma, to engage in deep connection with them when they share stories of abuse, violence, fear, and suffering. Empathy, that sensation of connecting to another's emotional experience, is one of the most common characteristics of most psychotherapists. It does, however, mean that we are exposing ourselves to vicarious trauma. Master therapists find ways to translate traumatic contagion into a more profound level of compassion. Experienced therapists who work with trauma survivors consistently report that they live more fully, treat others with greater kindness and respect, are more connected emotionally, and feel a greater sense of personal presence and strength (Kottler, 2017, p. 75). It is inspiring to me to learn how a patient managed to survive a violent encounter or help others during a crisis. I remind myself that I am working with survivors, not victims.

As I'm writing this book, we are in the midst of the COVID-19 crisis and attention has turned to the effects on health care workers of extended trauma in working with such a large number of very ill and dying patients. Regardless of our skill and level of training, we aren't prepared for the onslaught of human suffering brought on by health crises or natural disasters. Being immersed in fear and loss for weeks or months on end takes a toll. Those of us in working with emotional and mental disorders will also be engulfed by this pandemic as we reach out to those medical professionals, survivors, and the loved ones of those who die. The need will be overwhelming and I'm trying to prepare myself because I believe that the need for psychological services will be prolonged and massive on a global level. My experience working with 9-11 first responders will pale in comparison with the need as we begin to stabilize from this COVID-19 pandemic. We will be faced with all the grief, despair, and anger that accumulated with no real outlet for expression: No funerals, religious services, community gatherings, or other resources for expression of feelings and the comfort of others. Meeting this challenge will take a toll on therapists because of traumatic contagion coupled with our own losses and anxieties. Forming support groups with peers is my main focus at present as we begin to answer the calls for help.

Know Your Laws and Ethics (And Abide by Them)

Our ethical guidelines are there to protect both the patient and us. When in doubt about what to do, consult with supervisors or senior clinicians and take their advice. Know your ethical standards and follow them. In 40 years, I've never seen a good outcome for professionals who decide they can step outside of our ethics code. There's a good reason for each of the standards to be in place and if you aren't aware of the rationale for one of the standards, look up the research or consult with your professional organization. Unacknowledged needs on the part of psychotherapists for love, attention, and intimacy become a formula for disaster. Those entering the profession tend to minimize the degree of risk that they would ever become engaged in social or romantic relationships or manipulate patients for their own gratification. I share with them that I have had several colleagues and supervisors who are no longer in the profession because they engaged in an affair with a client, abandoned their family, and lost their license to practice. One, in fact, was the "star" of a PBS Frontline documentary titled, "My Doctor, My Lover" (https://www.pbs.org/wgbh/frontline/film/my-doctor-my-lover/, 1991).

Engage in Consistent Self-Care

In addition to taking care of our mental health and professional well-being, we need to pay attention to the basics: Eat well, get enough sleep, exercise regularly (my biggest challenge), and engage in routine health care. Your mind can only do its work if your body is well. Keep yourself healthy by doing healthy things. Get outdoors, take a walk, play with a child, read a good book, take a vacation, make something useful or lovely for yourself or someone else, get plenty of sleep, and eat a healthy diet. "Never operate a chain saw or do therapy without a good night's sleep" (Pipher, 2016, p. 74). If we believe in what we're doing to help others then we, to the best of our abilities, need to do it too.

I feel the effects of sitting in my office on the days that I see 8 or more patients. My body suffers from sitting all day and I need to get up and move around once I'm done before I settle in for the night. Even a 10-minute walk in the neighborhood or working for 20 minutes in the garden helps me feel refreshed and renew my energy. A brief yoga session helps work out the kinks from too much sedentary time and a brief session of meditation helps me transition to home and relaxing. I avoid junk food and sodas but drink lots of water. I am mindful about keeping regular physician and dentist appointments. If I'm ill, I stay home and rest. I can't encourage good health habits in others if I don't practice them as well.

Learn Something

I would add to the self-care list that having interests and activities outside of the profession is also an important aspect of self-care. I like to socialize with people who aren't psychotherapists. Every year, I make a point of learning something that I don't know much about. It's important to me to be a student again and to put my trust in someone who is teaching me something new. In the last ten years, I've learned to scuba dive, ride a motorcycle (my 65th birthday present to myself), make glass mosaics, cook in a cast iron skillet, and play dominoes among other things. It's refreshing to step out of the role of expert and do something interesting or fun that is novel for you.

Exploring new places, whether they are close to home or other countries and cultures, also engages our minds and reminds us there is a world outside the therapy office. I feel more energized and engaged when I'm in a new environment, particularly one that is unfamiliar. Even going to a restaurant that serves a type of cuisine I haven't tried before is a way to explore the unknown and learn something. Ethiopian food is marvelous! Reading a book written by someone from a different culture or background enlarges my world when I don't have the opportunity to travel. I read both fiction and nonfiction writers who offer a window into a population and environment that is unfamiliar to me.

Perhaps the most important thing is to step out of being in control and taking charge. Get out of the big chair and sit on the floor playing with Legos for a while. As a student of human behavior for nearly five decades, the one unbreakable rule that I'm aware of is that we can't learn less. When you work, work: When you play, play. Learn something new, whether through reading or doing, and have some fun along the way.

Connect to Other Therapists

Being a therapist means you have committed to become a life-long learner. Professional meetings, trainings and conferences also help to rejuvenate my love and devotion for my career. Inevitably, I hear someone speak or meet a colleague who inspires me to do better or to explore something different. I reconnect to the passion I have for this work and I fall in love with being a therapist all over again. I've had the opportunity to learn from so many wonderfully talented, creative, and compassionate therapists. I have a small tattoo on my left ankle of the Asian symbol for "Double Happiness. The symbol reminds me that the happiness we feel is doubled when we share it with others. I experience that increase in joy when I'm with others who love this profession as much as I do.

In addition to seeking therapy for ourselves, contact with colleagues is critical as both an outlet to talk about our dilemmas with patients and as a source of feedback about how we're functioning. Other therapists may help us see when our objectivity is compromised or when we're struggling to stay focused because of our own challenges. Supervision plays a vital role not just during our training and internships, but throughout our career. Ongoing consultation with other clinicians helps us gain perspective and improve our skills. Sitting down during a break with my colleagues at the office and just checking in with each other is another part of my self-care routine. I always find it a relief when I've been struggling with a difficult patient and one of my colleagues helps me change course and find a more effective way to work with them. Over the years, I have been fortunate to become friends with several of my colleagues and keeping in touch or visiting when we're able has been a delight. I've watched their lives change. We've shared our personal and professional success and listened to each other's heartbreaks. I am deeply grateful to have them in my life. Essentially, be sure you take care of your own mental health and relationships while you are working in this profession if you hope to have a long career.

Mindfulness

Another aspect of self-care that I find indispensable to my own mental health is mindfulness practice. I've studied Buddhism for more than 50 years and many of the practices and tenets of that philosophy have served me well both professionally and personally. My favorite definition of mindfulness is paying attention in a particular way: "…on purpose, in the present moment, and non-judgmentally" (Kabat-Zinn, 1994, p. 4). It's a remarkably helpful way to build unconditional positive regard and improve our self-awareness as therapists. Research has shown that therapists who practice mindfulness are better able to establish an empathic connection with their patients (Aiken, 2006). Learning to develop a calm focus and compassionate presence is well worth the effort; it impacts every aspect of our lives.

For me, meditation is happiness training, which is an essential part of my self-care. Meditation helps me stay more balanced and self-aware. I can usually tell I'm on to something good when the more I do it the better my life becomes. My daily gratitude meditation helps me maintain a more positive attitude and frequent, brief mindfulness exercises throughout the day keep me better focused, alert, and calm. There are hundreds of open access, online guided meditations and recordings of every sort as well as texts, trainings, and groups that are widely available. I encourage anyone unfamiliar with mindfulness practice to sample a variety of sources until you find one that feels comfortable. Some people like music with spoken word meditation, some don't; some want movement with the meditation (mindful walking), others want to sit still. There are endless variations and approaches, so explore and see what works best for you. The important thing is to make it a part of your daily routine so that's it becomes as important an aspect of self-care as brushing your teeth.

Lessons from the Big Chair: Chapter 7

- Have a life or you own and things you do aside from work.
- Know your Code of Ethics and follow it – no exceptions.
- Have at least 6 things that you can do to calm and care for yourself.

- Develop healthy habits for sleeping and eating.
- Learn something new on a regular basis.
- Practice mindfulness.
- Don't pretend that you're doing OK if you aren't. Get help for yourself.

Mindfulness Exercise

This is a brief meditation that I use at the beginning of a therapy session with some of my patients. I always invite them to join me but never require it. I like to introduce patients to a breathing meditation because it's a simple way to redirect our attention to something that is always with us, our breath. Several patients have made a recording of it that they use between sessions to help them focus or calm themselves. It's important not to rush and to time the directions to the patient's breathing pattern. Breathing along with the patient will give you a sense of their level of stress or comfort. I always instruct them that the mindfulness exercise will only take a few moments and that they are welcome to stop and just sit quietly at any time if they feel uncomfortable.

First, let's sit comfortably with our feet on the floor, hands in our lap or on our legs, and our eyes gently closed or looking softly at the floor. We are taking this opportunity to bring ourselves to this time we have together and to commit to being present with each other. We bring to this meeting our intention to speak openly and honestly and to listen to each other with compassion and respect. We become more present by focusing our attention on our breathing, breathing in through the nose and out through the mouth. Begin by noticing the rhythm of the breath, how it is cooler as it enters your body through the nose and warmer as it leaves your body. Just finding a comfortable rhythm that suits you as you breathe in….and out. Aware of the feeling of your chest gently rising….and falling. Aware of sounds in the room and outside, aware of thoughts or sensations you are having, but not needing to attend to anything other than your breathing. If you find your mind wandering, gently guide it back to your breathing, just as you would a small child who wanders away for a moment. Just return your focus to your breath.

With each breath, we can feel more centered, calm, and attentive. We breathe in a soft, golden light that comforts us....and breathe out any tension or discomfort that is in our body or mind. Breathing in the sparkling, golden light of kindness and compassion....breathing out tension and fear. Let us focus on the next 5 breaths with that image of filling ourselves with understanding and love when we breathe in and emptying ourselves of suffering and distress as we breathe out. (TAKE 5 BREATHS). As we become more relaxed and alert; we are ready to come together to create a better understanding, greater peace of mind, and a compassionate connection. When you are ready, take one more breathe and as you exhale, let your eyes gently open and we'll begin. Welcome.

PART III
HOW TO LET GO

The third big challenge that we all face is learning to let go. In Buddhist thought, suffering is caused by clinging to our current circumstance and resisting change which makes us unable to experience our life. All that we have we will eventually lose. Letting go, for most of us, is the most difficult thing we must learn as we go through life. This existential crisis is a common condition that brings people to therapy. Relationships, health, money, security, and everything else, including our lives, is impermanent. How we move through loss and change is the focus of this section.

Perhaps letting go is the biggest challenge because it's the one we don't look forward to. We must let go but we rarely want to and so we create suffering. The more we grasp, the more distress and unhappiness we experience. When we are faced with pain in our life, whether it's caused by a physical, mental, emotional, or interpersonal condition, our resistance or unwillingness to acknowledge and accept that pain is what creates suffering.

When people seek psychotherapy, it is usually because something very painful in their life has now become great suffering. We become locked in a struggle with an unbeatable foe. We insist that our life can't be what it is and so our painful experiences become battles within ourselves. "To let go is simply to release any images and emotions, grudges and fears, clingings and disappointments that bind our spirit" (Kornfield, 2008, p. 255).

There are three chapters in this section that focus on different aspects of learning to let go. The chapters are:

- **Chapter 8: Act or Accept?:** It is useful for therapists to understand problems that can be resolved through action and problems that require acceptance. We can't act our way out of being left behind when someone we love dies or leaves us or when we are facing catastrophic illness or injury. The chapter explores how we deal with moving toward acceptance of the unchangeable conditions we all face.

- **Chapter 9: Saying Goodbye:** This chapter explores an experience that is unusual for many of us; engaging in a positive end of an intimate relationship. The therapy relationship offers a rare opportunity to say goodbye in a meaningful way. As therapists, we learn to let go when our patients have made progress in meeting their goals. Creating a positive experience of saying goodbye can be very impactful for both patient and therapist.

- **Chapter 10: The End of Hope:** This chapter explores the experience of losing a patient who dies. Severe depression, drug addiction, eating disorders, domestic violence, and other problems can be fatal. This experience of "letting go" is the most challenging, difficult aspect of being in the big chair.

As psychotherapists, we are faced with learning to let go of patients who disappear, relapse, succumb to illness, are murdered or commit suicide. It is no small task to train our minds to experience the pain of losing a patient. It is, however, a task that we must embrace if we want a life in the big chair. Many who come into this profession either learn ways to cope with loss and let go or they change careers. This is the hardest part of what we do.

8

ACT OR ACCEPT?

The Talking Cure

For more than a century, we have pursued the "talking cure," psychotherapy, to address a long list of problems related to brain function, addiction, and behavioral, psychological, and emotional disorders. More than 3,000 research studies on the effectiveness of psychotherapy have demonstrated that there is a positive effect for patients, from children to the elderly, across a wide range of settings (Westra, n.d.). We know that psychotherapy helps many people in many ways. "Good therapy should rearrange the landscape of the mind" (Pipher, 2016, p. 36). It should help us be more authentic versions of ourselves, support us through challenging times, and help us connect to others more effectively and lovingly. On a pragmatic level, psychotherapy should also help us to not repeatedly make the same mistakes. Insanity is often described as doing the same thing over and over but expecting different results. For change to occur, something different must happen. The goal of psychotherapy is to help us become better people through making a difference in the patterns that create and perpetuate problems.

To become psychotherapists, we train for many years to learn the art and science of our craft. Throughout the history of our profession, psychotherapy training has largely focused on how to guide our patients in making behavioral changes. We have become adept at helping people learn to act differently and make more thoughtful choices in order to change their circumstances. Particularly in American culture, we embrace a "can do" approach to many of the problems that challenge us. Pipher (2016) sorted human problems into three categories: Those that can be solved through information and effort, those that require "sophisticated solutions" like psychotherapy, and those that are "simply not solvable" (p. 70). Psychotherapy, as we know it, is especially good at teaching clinicians to deal with the first two categories. Behaviorists, cognitive, and family therapy practitioners are particularly adept at providing information and developing complex strategies to motivate or instigate change, whether it's designing a reward system to reinforce more adaptive behavior patterns, teaching patients to think differently about their circumstances, or helping family members learn to interact more effectively. We have developed numerous pragmatic and effective approaches to problem solving for many of the challenges that we face.

Action Approach

Action strategies focus on making quantifiable changes in some aspect of our typical patterns whether it's changing a behavior, a thought, a mood, or an interaction. Action-oriented psychotherapy focuses on *doing* something different. The goal is to reduce our suffering by helping us to think, feel, and act in a manner that is more adaptive and creates a better result. Many of our problems can be improved or resolved by making a commitment to try a new approach to what we experience. We learn to exert control over ourselves and do something different to achieve a more favorable experience. Losing weight through diet change and exercise involves deciding to change how we eat and to become more active. We make cognitive and behavioral changes that lead to a more desirable outcome. If I stop telling myself that the person who just broke up with me was "the ONE," I will probably begin to feel better sooner. When I decline from watching horror movies before going to bed, I'll sleep better. Speaking calmly to my partner rather than yelling at him when I'm upset will probably improve our relationship.

Action therapies are also mind based; they focus on our ability to make choices about how we act and react. They require a commitment to undertake and maintain new patterns of thinking and behaving. In most situations, we can learn to be more aware of our responses and make choices about whether, when, and how to act. Viktor Frankl's (1959) "Man's Search for Meaning" is a poignant and elegant book about how, even in the worst of circumstances, we can choose our course of action. Frankl was interned as a prisoner of war by the German army during World War II. He observed that even in Nazi concentration camps, prisoners could choose to be predatory or compassionate. They could take advantage of the suffering of others or strive to ameliorate it. There are circumstances when everything can be taken from us but our ability to choose how we will react. Behavioral change is what we're good at as therapists, and it's effective with so many of the dilemmas we encounter, but it doesn't work for everything. There are circumstances and events that are beyond our control that we must learn to live with.

Acceptance Approach

An acceptance approach to therapy is something that all therapists must learn to do, but it is rarely a focus in training clinicians. Therapists are often called upon to assist patients in learning to accept things that they can't do anything about, and it seems that's an important skill for us to develop. I like the definition of acceptance as "…a willing movement of the heart, to include whatever is before it…" (Kornfield, 2008, p. 103). As we mature, we become more aware that our ability to change our circumstances has its limits. Everyone is confronted by experiences that we can't control. We are faced with events and changes that we didn't choose and can't stop. Approaching that type of problem with the focus on changing our thoughts or behaviors so that we can eliminate the unwanted experience simply won't work. There are times when we are faced with sad and painful issues that we can't think or feel or act our way out of. It goes back to Pipher's (2003) "simply not solvable" category of problems – those that we can't act our way out of or avoid.

Buddhism sees suffering as an expected and ordinary part of life; something that we all face. For some experiences, suffering is inevitable, as when we are terminally ill or a loved one has forsaken us. We must all learn to endure experiences that can't be changed. For this type of problem, the only cure is acceptance. Acceptance doesn't mean that we can't try to improve our circumstances, but we learn to understand that "just now, this is what is so" (Kornfield, 2008, p. 102). Psychotherapist Jon Carlson observed that "Sometimes I wonder if therapy isn't counterproductive when we encourage people to change anything they don't like instead of increasing tolerance for pain and greater acceptance of things outside of one's control" (Kottler & Carlson, 2014, p. 4). I agree with his concern. I believe that helping people learn how to accept and cope with what we can't change is an equally important approach to all the behavioral change skills that we typically focus on as therapists. Linehan (2020) incorporated her Zen Buddhist training to develop Dialectic Behavior Therapy, an approach that balances "acceptance or oneself and one's situation in life, on the one hand, and embracing change toward a better life, on the other" (p. 8).

A part of our training needs to teach therapists how to endure the unavoidable and to help others do so. How do we help our patients and ourselves to assess situations realistically, do what we can, and accept what we must? "The capacity to tolerate pain and sorrow is an underappreciated virtue" (Pipher, 2003, p. 71). Living with suffering and loss is a skill that we all must develop if we're to live a fully realized life. Patients who relentlessly focus on complaints about circumstances that they can't change create suffering out of their pain. Complaining about the unfairness of our partner leaving us or about a disability we acquired through an accident won't improve either that circumstance or our level of suffering, just the opposite.

Any therapist who's been in the big chair for a while has encountered patients who have arranged their lives and even their identities around unsolvable problems. They are stuck in complaints about not being treated fairly or not deserving the illness or issues that plague them. While I think it's important for us to vent about what has happened to us and express our outrage or sadness, over time that becomes an indulgence that hurts us. If we are trying to be something we are not, we exhaust our mind and body in a losing battle. Acceptance allows us to focus on the facts that we are faced with; to understand things just as they are.

The Importance of Learning Acceptance

Trying to solve a problem that's unsolvable creates more misery. There are the experiences that must simply be borne- loss and bereavement, sickness or disability, the decline of old age, and facing our own death. Unsolvable problems are not problems, they are life experiences. To manage painful life experiences, we must learn to change our focus. It's not so much what we can do, it's more about what we can be. Can I learn to be a person with diabetes? Can I be a mother whose son has died? Learning how to accept the unavoidable or inevitable allows us to awaken to our true selves. We can begin to develop some dignity and grace in accepting our life as it is and we can learn to incorporate the unwanted experience and bear it with compassion for ourselves and for others.

Accepting our life as it is and ourselves as we are move us to a greater sense of peace. "The only thing worse than feeling pain is not feeling pain" (Pipher, 2003, p. 54). Trying to avoid the unavoidable diminishes us; learning from the inevitable pain that life brings keeps us healthy. We need to know how to accept ourselves and how to help others do so as well. Inevitable experiences become more bearable when we don't resist them. I regret the times earlier in my career when I'm sure I made some patient's suffering worse by encouraging false hope: "Your husband will regret leaving you," "The doctor may have misdiagnosed your illness," "Your miscarriage was very sad, but I'm sure you'll be able to have a healthy baby." While I am a strong advocate of helping people find hope in their darkest times, I think that unrealistic hope simply pours salt in the wound. In some situations, hope is not about changing our circumstances, it's about changing or willingness to accept our life as it is.

Distinguishing Between Act and Accept

Being able to distinguish what constitutes a problem that can be addressed through action or through acceptance is part of the challenge. Certainly, our patients usually come in with the hope that we will help them find a way to reduce or eliminate their suffering, not help them learn to tolerate or even embrace it. The wish that seeing a therapist will make the problem go away or that we'll learn some secret about how to avoid our pain is not unusual. We want a Wizard who can make it all okay. The Serenity Prayer, a cornerstone of Alcoholics Anonymous (2001), provides an excellent guide to assessing the type of problem we are facing: "God grant me the serenity to accept the things I cannot change, the courage to change the things I can, and the wisdom to know the difference"(p. 41). Wisdom and the ability to distinguish between problems that can be solved and those that require acceptance is a skill that therapists would do well to develop. Understanding what type of problem we are facing helps us avoid a lot of useless "doing" and lets us focus more on "being." Assessing whether the approach in psychotherapy focuses on action or acceptance is helpful if we are to work toward a useful outcome.

There are several factors to consider when determining whether action or acceptance is the path. First is understanding "Who is your patient?" I'm often faced with patients who are trying to change something that they have no control over which usually involves attempting to change what another person is doing. If only their partner would be more like them, they would be happy. If their mother would just acknowledge what an abusive parent she was, it would free them of the anger they carry. Unfortunately, the partner and mother aren't the ones sitting in the office with me. Unless the other person is interested in joining us for sessions, there's not much we can do to influence them. When a patient is stuck in "if only….," the first task for a therapist is to help the patient wake up to the fact that "…it is they themselves who are inadvertently creating the unwanted situation and to stop doing it" (Claxton, 1999, p. 104). They are hoping for something that may be hopeless and is certainly out of their control. I will sometimes ask what is keeping them hopeful that the other person will change? Is there any evidence that the other person is interested in changing? How long do they want to wait to see if someone else would like to change? What is the impact on their life while they wait?

I find it productive to work with the person who is actually sitting in the office with me rather than trying to figure out anyone else's behavior or motives. I know how tempting it is to try and come up with a grand scheme that would allow the patient to do or say something that would fix their loved one, but it's a fool's errand. I often see novice therapists get locked into a "why don't you…," "have you tried to…" loop that is focused on figuring out what the patient can do that will change someone else or some unavoidable circumstance. It's an impossible task. I've never seen a good outcome from throwing suggestions at a patient that are designed to change another person. For anything of value to happen in therapy, it's important we help patients accept that they can only make changes in their own lives, not anyone else's.

Al-Anon, the support resource for loved ones of an addict, has spent decades helping people understand they are powerless to change an addict's behavior. Instead, they focus on how to accept and more effectively cope with what the addict is doing so that the member can reduce their own stress and disconnect from pursuing an impossible goal. Members learn instead to pay attention to their life and well-being, to prioritize what they need to do to be more functional and to let go of pursuing the addict to change. Paradoxically, that is sometimes the most effective strategy in getting an addict into treatment. When those who love them no longer make excuses for an addicts' behavior or try to prevent them from experiencing the consequences of their actions, it can get the attention of the person suffering from addiction by making it much harder to continue abusing substances.

When I'm working with a patient whose goal is to change someone else, it's always a reminder to me that I'm not there to change anyone else either. My goal is to help the patient make their own choices and determine their unique path. It's an odd paradox that therapists may have a much clearer perspective than anyone else on the impossibility of making another person change. We constantly experience that reality. People come to us expecting a bit of wizardry and get Dorothy instead. It's a bit of deception that we present ourselves as change agents when our real task is to convince patients that they, in fact, are the agent of change.

I use the following list to help determine whether a patient's dilemma will best be addressed through action or acceptance. The paradox, of course, is that acceptance is also a choice that must be acted on.

Action	Acceptance
Mind	Heart
Doing	Being
Action	Stillness
Commitment	Awareness
Control	Let Go

Mindfulness and Acceptance

Mindfulness approaches are effective in helping an enormous number of people by teaching us to become more aware of how our thoughts are creating our experience. Mindfulness has been described as "focusing attention, being aware, intentionality, being nonjudgmental, acceptance, and compassion" (Hick & Bien, 2008, p. 5). Meditation practices, on which mindfulness approaches are based, have been used in many parts of the world for more than 2,500 years. Psychotherapy and mindfulness practice are highly effective partners, particularly when we are dealing with problems related to acceptance.

Mindfulness training helps us learn to pay attention to ourselves and others "on purpose, in the present moment, and non-judgmentally" (Kabat-Zinn, 1994, p. 4). The heart of mindfulness is learning to be in the present moment and to become more connected to what is happening in our life and our thoughts. By attending to that inner voice that is evaluating our experience, we can establish a dialogue that nurtures awareness, clarity, and acceptance of our reality. "Mindfulness is the practice of directing our attention to only one thing. And that one thing is the moment in which we are alive" (Linehan, 2020, p. 280–281). The practice teaches us to step out of our critical evaluation of experience and witness the drama and comedy of our lives without drowning in it. It's not unusual for me to have a good laugh at myself when I am meditating. As we learn to embrace our experience and get on better terms with ourselves, it is easier to assist others in doing so.

Both patients and therapists can benefit enormously from learning mindfulness practices. For therapists, it can help expand compassion, develop a better sense of presence in therapeutic relationships, help us cope with stress, and reduce burn-out (Wheat, 2005). Developing a mindfulness practice can reduce levels of anxiety and depression, increase empathy (including self-acceptance), help to maintain cognitive clarity, and establish a greater capacity for tolerating discomfort (both physical and emotional). There are many approaches to developing mindfulness, but all of them teach us to be very attentive to how our thoughts, perceptions, and desires arise and how to catch our experience as it is being formed. I sometimes recommend Vishen Lakhiani's (2013) "6 Phase Guided Meditation" as a place to start for those who haven't practiced meditation. It's a brief (20 minutes) guided meditation that focuses on developing compassion, gratitude, forgiveness, vision for the future, control and support. It's available through YouTube at: https://youtu.be/EaRu14P9H84 . I've also become a fan of "Headspace", an on-line/phone app that has a wide variety of different formats and levels for those interested in learning or expanding their mindfulness practice.

An important aspect of acceptance is being able to tolerate the pain that is always part of the process of healing. It's why all good therapists keep an ample supply of tissues in their office. I make sure I have a box for my patients and one for myself. The yellow brick road leading to acceptance is filled with sadness, hurt, fear, and distress. In our culture, eliminating or avoiding pain as quickly as possible promotes additional distress when we are faced with painful circumstances that we can't escape. Suffering is seen as an aberration rather than a normal part of existence. Unhappy in your marriage? Get a new partner. Don't like your job? Leave. Feel tired, lonely or bored? There's a pill for that. The more we try to avoid or ignore negative life experiences, the more distressed we become. Ultimately, we must learn to face out fears and hurts, our traumas and problematic choices. No matter where you go, there you are.

Perhaps the best time to learn mindfulness practice is when we are faced with a problem that is simply not solvable. Although I had studied and practiced meditation from time to time since the age of 16, it was when I was confronted, at age 56, by my second husband's request for a divorce that I become serious about developing a consistent mindfulness practice. Since he was clear that he had no interest in attempting to reconcile, my only choice was acceptance. I wanted to learn to come to terms with the experience with as much grace and good-will (both toward him and myself) as I possibly could. Learning to stay present with the hurt, fear, and anger that I felt, rather than avoidance or pursuing distractions, was a difficult lesson to learn. My meditation sessions were very damp, I cried every day for many weeks. But, letting myself feel that pain and even embrace it let me move through the experience and emerge with a better understanding of myself, my ability to forgive, and the grace of letting go. I also developed a renewed appreciation for mindfulness practice. It was one of the most important experiences I've had and one that I have a deep appreciation for. Acceptance was the key to staying grounded and it helped me to build compassion both for my ex-husband and myself.

Don't Just Do Something, Sit There

We are all transformative beings, whether it involves taking action to make changes or learning to accept ourselves or, more likely, some of both. A colleague once shared with me that the best way to capture a monkey in the wild is to fill a hollow in a tree with ripe fruit. The hole in the tree must be just big enough for the monkey to get its hand in to grab the fruit, but not big enough for the monkey to withdraw its hand once it's holding the food. The monkeys that are trapped hang on to the fruit at the expense of their freedom. His kindness in sharing that story helped me decide to let go of a relationship that had me feeling trapped in a destructive pattern. There are stories that have the power to inspire and transform us and it's especially powerful when we become the hero of our story instead of the villain or victim.

Building a better foundation for acceptance of our experiences allows us to make choices that are in our best interest. "In letting go, even momentarily, of problem solving, possibilities emerge and, paradoxically, change becomes possible at just the moment we let go of change as a necessity" (Hick & Bien, 2008, p. 94). When we build a better connection to our inner experience and process, we have a deeper appreciation for what is happening in our lives and a greater sense of what we bring to situations and decisions. Our motives and desires, biases and beliefs are more accessible and not as likely to determine, without our consent, how we react to events and interactions. Mindfulness helps us learn to let go, to forgive, and to just be where we are in life. With practice, we can become adept at connecting to that calm inner core even when it feels like the eye of a hurricane.

Acceptance can be a hard sell for patients and therapists. It can seem as though we're giving up rather than waking up. I find, however, that letting go of struggling to change something, even for a little while, and sitting quietly at that "still point between action and nonaction" (Hick & Bien, 2008, p. 91) lets me feel calmer, freer, and more focused. There are some fights that we can't win, some things that we can't undo, and times that life will hurt like hell. The pain will be there, but the suffering can be reduced if we learn when to let go.

Lessons from the Big Chair: Chapter 8

- There are "problems" that are simply not solvable. If there's nothing one can do that would provide a solution, it's probably not a problem, it's a fact of life.

- Action therapies are mind based; they focus on our ability to make choices about how we act and react. They require a commitment to make and maintain new patterns of thinking and behaving.
- Acceptance therapies are heart based; they focus on times when we are faced with sad and painful issues that we can't think or feel or act our way out of.
- Living with suffering and loss is a skill that we all must develop if we're to live a fully realized life.
- Acceptance allows us to focus on the facts that we are faced with; to understand things just as they are.
- For anything of value to happen in therapy, it's important we help patients accept that they can only make changes in their own behavior, not anyone else's.
- Ultimately, we must learn to face our fears and hurts, our traumas and problematic choices. No matter where you go, there you are.
- Building a better foundation for acceptance of our experiences allows us to make choices that are in our best interest.

Case Study: Mandy

Mandy and I met following a referral from her physician. She was a 42-year-old, married, Hispanic woman who was the mother of two children. I worked with Mandy intermittently for over five years. There were periods of more intense therapy where we meet weekly and times when months would go by that I didn't hear from her. In her late 30s, she began to experience very severe head and neck pain. She would become immobilized for days, had to stop driving, and eventually lost her job. Despite several years of tests and assessments with numerous physicians, a definitive diagnosis was never made. The symptoms of her disorder changed a vigorous, successful, engaging, and competent woman into an invalid. Although she had a very caring husband and children who were devoted to her, she felt enormous guilt, anger, and frustration. She struggled with "why?" "Why was this happening to me? Why couldn't the doctors come up with a diagnosis and treatment plan? Why do I have to suffer?" Mandy was locked in a battle to return to her previous life. She was determined to get well and be the career woman, athlete, mother, and wife that she had been. For the first three years of our work together, that was her mission; to be her former self again.

Her reality was that she continued to become more incapacitated and restricted in what she could do. Everything she enjoyed in life – walks on the beach, making jewelry, running, traveling- were taken from her by the pain. Although there was no definitive diagnosis, it was determined she had a chronic, progressive, neurological disorder. The rage she had about being inflicted with the illness consumed her. She was sure that there was something that she and her doctors could do to defeat "the invader." The disorder was her enemy. She saw it as an intruder that had no right to interfere with the life she had planned. Mandy refused to accept what was happening to her. Often her attempts to act as if she didn't have the disorder led to exacerbations of her pain that incapacitated her for days or weeks.

It appeared to me that Mandy was determined to act her way out of her dilemma. When I tried talking with her about what it might mean to accept her life as someone with a serious disability, she became upset with that idea and made it clear to me that she wanted support for her goal of defeating the invader. Until the disorder appeared, she had been able to overcome many hardships by her determination and efforts. She had been in an abusive first marriage that she left, she had two children that she raised on her own while attending college and working, and she worked her way up to an executive position in a large company and earned a good living. She knew how to "do something" but not how to "sit there." What the illness demanded was the opposite of what had always worked best for her.

After a 6-month absence from therapy at the end of year four, Mandy called again for an appointment. Her goal of living without the pain began to shift to learning to live with the disorder. Her doctors had concluded that she had a complicated, progressive neurological disorder for which there was no available treatment other than pain management. After more than four years, Mandy was finally willing to accept that the invader was now a resident. We worked on acceptance and how to make her life fulfilling as the person she now was. Together, we said goodbye to her former self, studied mindfulness approaches to improve her pain tolerance, and focused on what she could do rather than what she couldn't. It was a slow process; letting go takes time.

I continue to talk with Mandy about once a month, usually by phone since she has days when she can't walk very well or ride in a car. When she has good days, she comes to the office and we celebrate her ability to get out of the house. I keep a box of tea that she likes for us to share. She discovered the joy of audiobooks, she chooses recipes for her husband and older daughter (both of whom love to cook) that she would like to try, and she Skypes with friends and relatives so that she doesn't feel so isolated. She's living the life that she has now. I'm very proud of her.

Lesson from the Big Chair: Acceptance

Mandy embodies the struggle that we all face when we encounter life changes that we don't want and can't avoid. Letting go of the hope that we can go back to time when we could overcome obstacles and determine our fate is a painful struggle. It is one that we all are likely to face at some point. Mandy helped me appreciate the courage it takes to move from action to acceptance. While we can't avoid pain, we can impact the degree of our suffering by examining how to live the best life we are able to regardless of our circumstances. By not letting go of a dream that we can't manifest, we lose what joy or peace we might have in life. Like Mandy, I hope to have the wisdom to know the difference between what I can and can't do.

9

SAYING GOODBYE

Letting Go

Letting go is the third lesson that we must learn as human beings. Perhaps it's the last on the list because it is the most challenging for most of us. I believe it's a part of clinical training programs that is sometimes over-looked, sadly so because it can be such a poignant yet healing part of the therapeutic relationship. We talk about "termination" but not so much about saying goodbye. It's a treasured experience for me because it's a rare opportunity. A planned end to therapy gives both the patient and me a chance to experience "a positive conclusion in what might have been a life-time of negative, unresolved, or empty endings." (Gottlieb, 2019, p. 353). We typically remember our relationships based on how they came to an end. It's such a gift for me to say goodbye to a patient who has made progress and send them off to a life that better suits them, one that is more authentic and fully realized. It feels unfair sometimes that when "we feel comfortable and safe, when we even look forward to the meetings with clients we have grown attached to, it is time to say goodbye" (Kottler, 2017,

p. 90). A positive ending to a therapy relationship is a memorable experience, hopefully for both of us.

Meaningful goodbyes are one of the most wonderful and informative parts of being a psychotherapist. Termination (a term I dislike, it sounds rather brutal) can offer a chance to gather important information about what the client found most helpful, encourage continued progress, discuss ongoing resources for support or assistance, and to have a positive end to the relationship. Having closure through a mutually agreed on and compassionate end to our therapy relationship is a rare opportunity given how often intimate relationships of any kind end badly. I hope that anyone working in this field has the chance to experience the type of goodbye that is "...the emptiest and yet the fullest of all human messages..." (Vonnegut, 1987).

Throughout the course of therapy, I intermittently bring up the question, "How will we know when our work here is done?" In our first meeting, I ask that question to set the expectation that we will only travel so far together and that we have a goal we are working toward. I sometimes remind patients that our purpose is not to grow old together, it's for them to transform to a closer approximation of the person they want to be. That question also helps me keep focused on what is important about the work we're doing together. Having a clearer sense of what to watch for lets both of us know when we are finishing what we've come together to accomplish.

Formulating treatment plans is an integral part of training in all therapy disciplines and is embedded in the requirements for most agencies, clinics, and hospitals that provide psychotherapy. Treatment plans evolve throughout the course of therapy and offer a flexible map of the territory to be explored. Treatment plans ought to include the question of what our expectations are for termination. I ask patients in our first meeting, "If this were our last session together, what is different about you?" I want them to begin to form an image of the person they want to be through their involvement in therapy. I also want to keep that image of who they will be at the end of therapy as a guide for what to watch for in sessions. If a patient wants to be less isolated after his wife's death and start meeting more people, hearing him talk about getting involved in volunteer work at the library and having lunch with other volunteers lets me know that we're moving toward a successful end to our work.

In all relationships, the end is embedded in the beginning. In marriage, we vow to remain connected "until death does we part." In therapy, we stay connected until the patient has become empowered and achieved an acceptable resolution to their concerns. As Yalom (2017) states, "Psychotherapy is not a substitute for life but a dress rehearsal for life…though psychotherapy requires a close relationship, the relationship is not an end – it is a means to an end" (p. 182). Empowerment and emancipation, not dependence, are what I watch for in patients. I'm always mindful that the primary goal of therapy is for the patient to no longer need me.

When to Let Go

Knowing when to end a therapy relationship is as important as knowing how. Although a treatment plan offers a guide for determining the completion of the patient's specific goals, there are several unstated goals that I watch for. I look for an increase in their compassion, both for themselves and others. Are they able to claim their humanity and recognize it in others? Have they learned to be kind to themselves and accept their fallibility and uniqueness? Can they be gentle with themselves when they are struggling? As Pipher (2016) notes, "To survive, we must all learn to live in the world with broken hearts" (p. 176). Successful therapy doesn't mean we are free of suffering, it means we are able to better incorporate it in our journey. Are they able to accept that everyone has suffering in life and can they extend compassion to both themselves and those they encounter?

Gottlieb (2019) describes "…one litmus test of whether a patient is ready for termination is whether she carries around the therapist's voice in her head, applying it to situations and essentially eliminating the need for the therapy" (p. 355–356). Jim, a gentleman in recovery from drug addiction, told me after several months of working on relapse prevention that he was in a situation where he felt the urge to use and he heard my voice talking back to his "addictive voice" in support of his recovery. Almost everything that we learn we've incorporated from others who shared information or their experiences with us. We often hear it in our minds as the teacher's voice speaking to us for some time before it becomes a part of our own internal dialogue. When I hear a statement like Jim's, it's a signal that our work together has taken hold on a deeper, internal level. As that voice became his voice, he began to feel more confident and secure that he could confront challenges more independently.

Effective therapy is a process of letting go of aspects of ourselves that interfere with living a more authentic, empowered life. It's a lesson in letting go of the narrative that holds us back and traps us in a cycle of experience that diminishes who we are. I sometimes recommend to clients that they read Hans Christian Anderson's (1844) story "The Ugly Duckling." It can be particularly helpful if the client's narrative has been one of being born into a family or other circumstance (such as poverty or domestic violence) that convinced them they could not have the life they wanted and that they were flawed in some immutable way. Many of us must unlearn stories we were taught in order to recognize who we are. Most people have some piece of an "ugly duckling" they hold as the truth about themselves and it can be the focus of therapy to help them discover their true "swan" nature.

I also know it's time to begin the process of saying goodbye when our sessions become less focused and there's a sense of "I'm not sure what to talk about today" on the part of the patient. I often increase the time between sessions and give more homework for patients to focus on between our meetings as the therapy is coming to an end. I want to transfer the work they are doing from the office to their home. I'm typically more active at the beginning and end of the relationship. I feel it's my responsibility to set the guidelines in place for therapy sessions at the beginning (e.g., meeting times, payments, cancellation policy, etc.) and again at the end when they have progressed in meeting the goals they set. When I sense that the patient is ready to move on from our work together, I sometimes use a session to review the goals we set when we began our sessions. It's common for me to bring up the idea of ending therapy. I ask if they feel they have accomplished what they planned to through our work together and whether it's time to talk about saying goodbye? I want to involve the patient in the decision about when to end and to have time to address any unfinished business that might be left.

The Final Session

When I'm planning a final session with a patient, I ask them to think about what happened for them during our time together that was helpful and what made our work effective? Also, I ask them to think about anything that got in their way during our time together, anything that they found unhelpful. It's equally important for me to know both of those things. It's the type of feedback that is invaluable to guide our work and help us to be more effective and self-aware. I want to know what they learned during our work together, what lessons they are using to help guide their life going forward. Finally, I ask them to think about how they felt during our first meeting and how they feel about saying goodbye. It's important to spend time sharing the feelings of loss if this has been a significant experience that we've shared.

My goal during a goodbye session is to help the patient express their feelings and consolidate the gains they made and the lessons they learned. I hope they leave our last meeting feeling satisfied that they have progressed and learned things that are now a part of their approach to life. Effective therapy not only helps resolve the initial dilemma that brought someone through the door, it offers them an expanded and more useful set of skills for being in their world. It's the difference between giving someone a fish to eat and teaching her to fish. I hope that our work made it possible for the patient to have a better fit with their life, to be a more fully realized person whoever that may be for them. I believe that when we can lay claim to our life – our history, mistakes, achievements, gains and losses – it allows us to be better able to cope with and even embrace what lies ahead.

I prepare for our final session. I spend time remembering what the patient was like when they first came to see me, my thoughts, and impressions of them. I take time before the final meeting to get a clear image in mind of who they were when we first met. I want to share in specific terms how I see a difference since our first encounter. I may comment on how they appeared in the first few meetings, "I remember how hard it was for you to tell me about the experience that brought you here," and contrast that with what I see in them as we're concluding our work, "I see you as more open to new experiences and patient with yourself as you learn how to cope" The most rewarding experience I have in this profession is to see people become more of who they want to be. "We watch our patients let go of old self-defeating patterns, detach from ancient grievances, develop a zest for living, learn to love us, and, through that act, turn lovingly to others" (Yalom, 2017, p. 258).

It's equally important that I let them know how our work together has changed me. I let them know that I'm grateful for what they've shared with me. I often comment that "Our time together has made me appreciate how brave and determined you are in changing the course of your life. That has helped me feel more courageous and committed to making changes in my life." I thank them for that lesson and for the opportunity they offered me to change along with them. I also share what I found most hopeful and positive as well as what made our work challenging for me. If they have made progress in our work, I do feel differently about them than I did in our initial meetings. I'm more connected and appreciative of their determination to manage make important changes. Most importantly, I want to make sure that I'm Dorothy, not the Wizard. I was just a companion on their journey, not some powerful being who changed their life. The patient takes credit for the work done to transform their experience or learn to cope more effectively. Empowerment is always my goal in therapy, it's the "learning how to fish" lesson so that they can take better care of themselves. It's a bit like graduation; the student's efforts are acknowledged even though their teachers worked hard as well. It's the student who's celebrated and whose accomplishments are recognized.

Sudden Endings

Like our social and romantic relationships, goodbyes in therapy are more likely to be abrupt and unexplained. Many patients end therapy before the therapy is ended. Research indicates that a third of patients don't return after the initial interview and approximately half of all patients leave therapy after the first two sessions (Goldberg, 2012). One thing that those new to the profession need to understand is that you will be left wondering, "What happened?" much of the time. I find the experience is like being in an enormous library, filled with amazing, heartbreaking, inspiring stories. You pick up a book, open it to a random page somewhere near the middle, read a few pages or chapters and then close the book and put it away. You don't know enough of the story to know where it's going and that can be troubling.

I sometimes long to know whether former patients are doing better as a result of our time together. Did their choice to leave a relationship free them from abuse? Did going back to school open doors to a better life for them? Have they been able to find happiness again after a profound loss? One thing most experienced therapists develop is an enormous capacity to tolerate uncertainty. Unless a patient dies while in therapy, we never really know the end of the story. When a patient leaves therapy before we're finished with the work, I wonder what it was that took them out the door that last time? One thing that's missing is any opportunity for feedback or a chance for redemption if I did something that contributed to their decision to leave.

All psychotherapists must get used to feeling rejected. While no one enjoys that experience, for those of us who have personal struggles with rejection, it can be a particularly challenging part of our work. It's not too dissimilar to "being ghosted" when you are dating. You meet someone that you are interested in spending more time with and they seem interested in you, then they just disappear without explanation. Regardless of the type of relationship, that can be a challenging way to end and leaves unanswered questions or concerns.

I suspect that all therapists find some way to rationalize those rejections: "The patient wasn't ready," "They were too resistant," "They weren't motivated," or "There was some transference that the patient wasn't able to deal with." We all have our favorite fantasies about why the patient didn't come back that puts the responsibility squarely on their shoulders. In fact, it hurts to be rejected regardless of what type of relationship you have with someone. I often wonder how patients are doing when they leave therapy unexpectedly. I'm left trying to determine, "What happened?" "What did I do, or not do, that they didn't return?" It's especially heartbreaking when it's a patient with whom you've invested significant time and energy; someone who you feel hopeful for and see making progress. Sometimes, in reviewing my work with a patient who disappears, I get an idea about what I might have missed. Now, however, it's too late to do anything with that possibility. It's a frustration I always find hard to handle.

Many years ago, I gave up the practice of following up with a phone call when I had a no-show. Unless there is a reason for me to be concerned about their welfare, I find that most people simply avoid the call or are unwilling to share the reasons for their disappearance. If a patient is planning to come back, I'll hear from them. I also don't follow my patients on social media or keep in touch other than to respond to messages or contact from them. It seems invasive to me to monitor what's happening to patients on social media, rather like cyber-stalking a former friend. Because I know how much courage it takes to make that first step to set an appointment and go see a therapist, I'm sad when someone leaves without warning or explanation. You will have innumerable experiences of being confused and uncertain about what went wrong.

The most difficult of the patients who leave abruptly are those who may be in danger or at risk. When people disappear who are in domestic violence situations, potentially suicidal, homeless or living on the edge, or struggling with severe mental illness or substance abuse there can be a real sense that they may never be able to return. Despite our desire to know what has happened, we must live by laws and ethics regarding their confidentiality. This type of loss of a patient is certainly a common topic in supervision and with colleagues. I often have a mix of fear, sadness, and anger about being in the dark, especially if I believe there is a credible risk to them after they leave therapy. With high-risk patients, I will reach out if possible, with a call or text to see if they want to reschedule. I don't attempt to contact a patient when it's a domestic violence situation or other circumstance where it might endanger them if I try to follow up. Those are the patients who keep most of us up at night. It's not unlike what parents feel when their child is in trouble and avoiding contact. It's the hardest type of letting go; to be left with fears about a patient's well-being.

Time to Leave the Nest

The other side of the goodbye experience is the patient who doesn't want to leave. In our social and romantic relationships, most of us have, or will have, the opportunity to be both the one who leaves and the one who's left. Neither are enviable or pleasant experiences, but both can teach us a great deal about letting go. While it's much more common for the patient to initiate the end of therapy, there are times when the therapist must take the lead in ending the relationship and that is a difficult task at best. Therapy is rather like raising children. You create a loving, nurturing, warm relationship with your child with the goal of making them increasingly less dependent on you and more able to be functional in the world. Some patients, like some children, move themselves forward toward greater independence, some do not. For those who do not, the effort is required to push them out of the nest.

I'm always reluctant to initiate a termination with a patient who is not making any progress and tend to err on the side of waiting too long. My concern is whether it's a problem with trust and if more time and patience might be necessary for the work to be productive. I put effort into making a connection and exploring what I might be doing or not doing that could be keeping us stuck. The red flags for me are missed appointments and payments, patients who continually focus primarily on what other people in their life need to do, abbreviated sessions because the patient has "nothing to talk about," patients who don't follow through on commitments or assignments to which they have agreed, engaging in "small talk," and interrupting sessions to take phone calls or leave early.

I make clear to patients that I start and end sessions on time and that the hour I set aside is for them, just as the time before and after their appointment, is reserved for other patients. I ask that they put phones and other screens away while we meet so that we aren't distracted. It's rare for me to "fire" a patient, but after three sessions with a young woman who insisted on taking personal and work-related calls during our meetings (none of which were emergencies), I told her that she could reschedule with me in the future only if she agreed to turn off her phone. That was our last session together.

When I have a clear sense that the patient might be overly dependent, malingering, or have some other agenda (such as placating a spouse or appeasing an employer), I usually begin the dialogue by asking what benefit they're getting from our work? How is the therapy helpful to them? I also share my feelings about our relationship and that I find myself puzzled about what we are doing that is useful for them? I may share that I feel stuck or frustrated with our relationship, particularly if I seem to be working harder than they are. It's a delicate conversation and I always strive to focus on my feelings and reactions, not to blame the patient. There can be any number of factors that are getting in our way. There are common issues such as a complicated transference, staying in therapy to avoid a consequence (e.g., an ultimatum from a spouse or a court order), using therapy as a substitute for friendships, being dependent on the therapist, their friends are in therapy and they want to be too, or seeing the therapist as responsible for changing their life for them. If we can determine what is keeping them in therapy, we can sometimes have a meaningful talk that moves us forward. There are times, however, that I have to make the decision to end the relationship because what we're doing is not therapeutic.

To initiate termination with a patient who is not making appropriate use of our time together, I might space out meetings to every other week or once a month. Sometimes, more time between sessions is helpful in giving them time to think about their commitment to the process or address homework assignments that they have avoided. Once I have shared my concerns about their commitment to therapy and scheduled additional time between meetings to encourage them to consider whether they want to continue, I will initiate an end to therapy if they don't become more engaged in the process. I will schedule a final session with the patient for us to do an assessment and encourage them to return in the future or see if working with someone else is more useful for them. Damage assessment means that I share my frustration that I couldn't be of more help, that sometimes timing is important in making progress and now might not be the best time. I don't focus on the patient's behavior; I focus on my own thoughts and feelings. While I may not be able to help them, I certainly want them to have a positive ending so that they would not be reluctant to seek help from someone else in the future. Even when I initiate the ending, I still want to share my impressions with them and acknowledge any progress that they've made, even if it's simply their courage in coming to meet with me.

Lessons from the Big Chair: Chapter 9

- There is a positive effect for both patient and therapist in letting go of the relationship when the work is done.
- Letting go in a compassionate, meaningful way is a rare and valuable experience.
- Share with patients how the relationship with them has impacted and changed you and make sure they take credit for the work and changes they've made.
- Making peace with uncertainty and rejection are helpful to maintaining a career in the big chair.
- Sometimes, it is our job to push the bird out of the nest. Therapy is successful when it helps people have a better life, not be a better patient.
- Mindfully saying goodbye is a wonderful, sad, rare experience.

Case Study: Betty

Betty was a 50-year-old, divorced, white woman who was sent to me by her physician who had just prescribed antidepressants for her. When I met her in the waiting room, Betty had a large, brightly colored, quilted bag, a book, and a file of notes from her doctor. She wore large glasses that concealed most of a very pale face. When I extended my hand in greeting, she looked away and offered a very gentle handshake. When she came in to the office, she made little eye contact and sat very still in the middle of the couch hugging her large bag on her lap.

Betty had moved to Florida from the northeast three years ago when her 80-year-old mother was diagnosed with Alzheimer's. She was the youngest of four children; all other members of her family lived in New England. Betty's father had suffered a stroke that disabled him and he lived in assisted care near her mother's apartment. Betty was the caretaker for both of her parents. She had a very close relationship with her mother and was grateful to be living with her. She had left her job when she moved to Florida and her siblings helped provide financial assistance so she could devote herself to her parents.

We worked on her long history of anxiety which had led to her inability to return to work. Except for her relationship with her parents and some people at her mother's church, Betty was very isolated. She had been married once in her 20s to a man who was both physically and psychologically abusive to her. Since her divorce when she was twenty-five, she had no other intimate relationships and hadn't made any friends since her move to Florida. Her shyness and anxiety had always made it difficult for her to connect to others. True to her nature, she always asked how I was doing and expressed concern any time I had to be away from the office. She sometimes brought homemade cookies and small handmade gifts to decorate the office. She never missed an appointment unless it was an emergency with one of her parents.

During the time we worked together, her father died, Betty injured her leg and had to use a cane, her mother's condition deteriorated, Betty was put on disability (after more than a year of repeated assessments and denials), and finally, Betty's mother died. During the final year of her mother's illness, Betty developed a friendship with an employee at the apartment complex where she lived who frequently helped her bring in groceries and manage other chores that were difficult for her. The relationship became more intimate and when Betty's mother died, she and her friend decided to marry. They moved back to New England to be closer to her friends and family.

Our sessions were a series of processing losses and letting go. Everything that she was terrified of happened: She lost her parents, she became disabled and financially insecure, and she risked becoming intimate with a man. It was a long struggle to accept a life that she had been frightened of for decades. As her fears came to pass, however, her anxiety began to abate. She had enormous grief, but was less concerned about what the future held. She was able to find her way through all her losses with as much grace as anyone could hope.

Betty was an intelligent, thoughtful, kind woman who had put her own needs aside to care for her parents. Despite her own challenges, she was patient and compassionate with both her father and mother. She was willing to risk becoming intimate with a man, something she never believed would be possible for her. I came to greatly admire Betty. When it was time to set our final appointment before her move, I had to learn to let go. It had been such an inspiration to watch her approach her challenges with quiet determination and to witness the courage she developed during our time together.

In my goodbye to her, I shared my admiration of how far she had come in the two years we worked together. How she had changed from the lost, frightened soul that I first encountered to the woman who was creating a new chapter, one that I hoped would be the happiest part of her life story. I told her that she was one of my best teachers regarding compassion, patience, and kindness. I hoped that I would face my own fears with as much grace as she had shown. Betty showed me how living through what scares us the most has the potential to bring out what's best in us. I felt I had also become more loving and less fearful through our meetings. I thanked her for helping me and for giving me the opportunity to be of help to her. We embraced, said some tearful "goodbyes" and let go.

Lesson from the Big Chair: Letting go

It was hard to close Betty's story and put it on the shelf, but it's a story that stayed with me and inspires me still. Being able to stay connected on her journey through so much pain and loss was a gift to me. I often think of Betty with deep gratitude for what she taught me about letting go and for the grace and courage that she brought to our work together. Although we haven't had contact in the years since our work ended, I am hopeful that her life has continued to expand and that her loving presence has graced the lives of others as it did mine.

10

THE END OF HOPE

Letting Go of Hope

This last chapter on letting go is the most difficult to write because letting go of hope goes against my instincts and desires. Giving up hope is the hardest lesson of all that I've had to learn as a psychotherapist and as a human being. I'm sure that's why this chapter comes near the end of the book – I wanted to avoid immersing myself in the memories of failure, loss, and the sadness that is often a part of doing this work. Facing death is the final lesson in letting go; letting go of everything that we have and that we are. So many of the patients we serve are vulnerable to the tragedy of overdose, violence, terminal illness, and suicide. "Hope and despair are a therapist's constant companions" (Kottler & Carlson, 2014, p. 247). While we cling to optimism and hope for good outcomes for our patients, we must also learn to embrace our failures and limits. The hardest lesson is learning to confront our own despair and experience the grief of losing a patient.

Facing the impact of the COVID-19 pandemic has made it clear how important it is for mental health professionals to hone their skills in working with grief and loss. As I'm writing this in late April 2020, we are still experiencing increasing numbers of deaths every day all over the country. For many years to come, we will be helping others cope with the effects of this illness that is claiming so many lives and impacting families, health care professionals, and first responders. Almost no one will be the same after we emerge from this experience. For nurses, doctors, and others working to help those who are stricken, the degree of trauma is something we have only seen in combat situations and during other historic pandemics. Training in trauma-based therapies and grief counseling should no longer be an elective course of study or a specialty area. We know that working with those directly impacted by COVID-19 will also be traumatic for therapists as we hear the litany of loss. Undoubtedly, most of us will have direct experience of loss due to this illness or will suffer the effects ourselves. We will lose family members, friends, patients, students, colleagues, mentors, professors, and others just like everyone else. Building networks of support and layers of services for those affected and those providing psychotherapy to them is critical. We have a great deal of work to do.

When a Psychotherapy Patient Dies

When a patient dies from the effects of an addiction or a behavioral/psychiatric disorder, the enormity of what we do becomes much clearer. This work really is about life and death and not everyone makes it out alive. The impact of the disappearance or death of a patient is an experience that changes us. I often know my patients more intimately than my friends. I'm privileged to learn their secrets and hidden histories, sometimes I'm the only one who knows certain parts of their life story. I'm much more conscious of my vulnerabilities and how temporary life is for all of us. One day, I will run out of time and it will be my turn to die. I hope to be able to approach that day with as much grace, compassion, and peace of mind as possible. I also want that for the people I serve.

For me, the hardest aspect of being a psychotherapist is losing a patient. It's inevitable, however, that all of us who occupy the big chair will eventually go through that experience – probably several times over. Mental illness, like physical illness, can be terminal. Our patients die from the effects of their disorders and are often at higher risk for accidents, homicides, serious medical illnesses, drug overdose, and suicide or homicide.

We encounter many people who have lost hope. It never becomes easy or routine to sit with someone who sees no reason to live because their life has become so painful. At the time of writing this, we're also losing patients to COVID-19 and dealing with grief in isolation, as are the friends and family members of those who are dying. Not being able to have direct contact or offer comfort to someone we care about who is ill or dying is an enormous complication in our grief and one that we will have to develop a way to cope with effectively.

Early in my career, I met Gina, a 45-year-old woman with whom I met for several months. She had a long history of physical abuse and abandonment, decades of drug and alcohol addiction, and crippling anxiety and depression. Gina had recently been diagnosed with a particularly virulent form of cancer and her physician had recommended that she seek psychotherapy. In order to receive treatment for her cancer, she had to stop all drug and alcohol use which meant she was also experiencing withdrawal symptoms along with the side effects of her chemotherapy. She was sick, exhausted, and unable to sleep or eat. Her main source of relief, being intoxicated, was no longer available. She seemed to me like the character, Alex, in "Clockwork Orange" (Burgess, 1962) who was forced to watch a film of horrific events with his eyes pried open. Just as she was feeling her worst, there seemed to be no place in her life that offered her any relief or sanctuary; no highs, no sleep, no friends, or family nearby to comfort and care for her. Just spending an hour with her each week left me fatigued and shaken. I learned quickly to make her my last session of the day since I was in no condition to see anyone else after meeting with her. She was desperate for relief and had no idea what to do. I didn't know either.

With some patients, regardless of how much I dig through the shit, I'm unable to "find the pony." With Gina, it was hard to imagine an end to her misery or to find something positive or life-affirming in her suffering. The only thing I knew to do for Gina was to sit with her each week as she reviewed the litany of pain that was her life. I saw her for several months until she became too ill to continue with sessions. We had phone sessions after she moved away to live with a sister who cared for her and later when she was admitted to hospice. In the final few calls, we talked about dying and her fears and hopes. She talked about her anger at feeling she had wasted so much of her life and her hope that her suffering would soon be over. At best, I was someone who would just listen to her, not offer false hope or platitudes. I don't know that I was any help to her. She, however, was a help to me. Gina helped me learn to bear witness to another's suffering when all I could do was offer her the comfort of not being alone.

A Good Death

It is hard work to be with someone who is gravely ill or dying. It's inevitable that we see our own mortality reflected in them. "Sitting mindfully with our sorrows and fears, or with those of another, is an act of courage." (Kornfield, 2008, p. 99). An experience that I cherish is when a patient who is facing death is open to exploring how to have a "good death," one that minimizes suffering and helps them to be at peace with who they are and how they've lived. While it's a rare experience, I have been privileged to travel that path with several patients who transformed fear and anger to grace and peace as they let go of the struggles of life. I trust there will be more in the coming days as the pandemic continues.

Erikson (1980) described our task at the end of life as the struggle between integrity and despair. As we grow older, we tend to have fewer external demands from jobs and family. There is time to contemplate both our accomplishments and missed opportunities. When we have a greater sense of having a successful life, of having lived the life we wanted to live, there's a sense of integrity and satisfaction. I find myself increasingly grateful for the opportunities I've had to encounter so many remarkable people who entrusted me to join them on this final part of their path in life. If, however, we see our life as unproductive or feel that we did not accomplish our life goals, our dissatisfaction and regrets can lead us to despair. For some, the cost of not following our heart is spending our later years wishing we had. The challenge in confronting despair is becoming willing to accept the past as it is and let go of regrets.

While our work focuses on helping people have a better life, I think we must also prepare to help our patients have a better death. Clinicians can reduce depression, if it arises, in end-of-life matters, as well as other mental health problems associated with pending death. We can also support caregivers and family members with facilitating emotional expression and becoming good listeners for people who are dying (American Psychological Association, 2005). I find that the work with dying patients often focuses on forgiveness and compassion, for themselves and others, and gratitude for their life. The goal of therapy becomes helping patients to approach their death with fewer regrets and a greater acceptance of the totality of their life experience. Sometimes there's a chance to make amends and provide or seek forgiveness or share toxic secrets that have been harmful. Creating greater peace of mind when we are dying can mean unburdening ourselves of resentments and regrets, grudges and hostilities. We can come to accept ourselves as the fallible, vulnerable, imperfect beings that we are.

In a meta-analysis of studies about people's desires regarding their death, the top three concerns were the dying process (having good conditions such as dying in their sleep or in a familiar, comfortable environment), being pain free, and their emotional well-being. The study also noted that "there is a dearth of research examining the psychological aspects of a good death, particularly from a patient perspective" (Meier, Gallegos, Thomas, Depp, Irwin & Jeste, 2016). We can assist our patients with many tasks such as making peace with others in their lives, letting go of resentments and unfulfilled desires, alleviating fears about dying, leaving something mean-ingful for others, and a range of other things that can offer greater peace of mind. Most importantly, we can be a compassionate witness and listen to them without interruption or judgment. For family and close friends, listening to their loved one talk about death can be uncomfortable and that discomfort often keeps dying people silent. They don't want to add any more difficult emotions to the experience for themselves or others.

Regardless of the age at which we are faced with our imminent death, the acceptance of our feelings of satisfaction and regret is still there. We want to make our exit with some grace and good-will, without too much fear and pain. A sudden, unexpected death deprives us of the opportunity to assess and embrace the life lived. We're denied the chance to explore: Did I live well? Love well? Will I be remembered by others with affection or disdain? Was my life determined primarily by fear or love? Am I leaving anything of value for others? Has the impact of my life been more helpful than harmful? What have a learned that I want to share with others? An anticipated death gives us the chance to embrace what our life has been and let go.

A Bad Death

I have also been a witness to people who are filled with rage or terror as they face death. It seems that how we approach dying often reflects how we approached living. Lives that are filled with fear can lead to terror at the end. Letting go is the hardest of the three tasks we must learn in life and not all of us die with grace. Becker (1973) observed that the fear of death must be present to motivate us toward self-preservation, yet we also tend to remain oblivious to this fear in our daily life. We know that there was a time before we existed and there will be a time when we cease to exist, but that is a reality that we tend to ignore. In many cultures including ours, dying is seen as something to fear and to overcome through religious belief. For example, Christianity focuses on overcoming death through faith that our spirit will continue to exist even when our body dies. There is a denial of the finality of death in the belief that you can live forever and reunite with loved ones if you are a believer. There is certainly a consequence to nonbelievers who will suffer endlessly in hell after they die, a pretty frightening concept.

Buddhist practice requires us to deliberately face our death and meditate on the reality that each moment could be our last. Meditation on death is a path to becoming more at peace with impermanence and the reality that there was a time before me and there will be a time after me. In Thich Nhat Hanh's book, "No Death, No Fear" (2002), he focuses on the illusion of birth and death and that "coming and going are just ideas" (p. 194). It's a book that I often recommend to people who are struggling with a fear of death. He writes about the nature of impermanence and interconnectedness and how a deeper understanding of these realities can lower our anxiety. While there are many paths to making peace with death, it is an important part of our work to find a way to bring a calm, loving presence to those who are dying. We can't be afraid to face death if we are to help others through that experience. If we are avoidant or fearful about death, we will amplify the suffering of others who are also frightened.

Sitting in the big chair requires us to become adept at talking about subjects that are often avoided in social conversation: Sex, violence, drug use, and death. For me, it's taken a lot of practice to build a level of comfort in discussing illness and death with patients. As I'm getting older and confronting my own mortality, I've become more open to having the "existential crisis" conversation with patients. I always have several patients who are coping with serious, chronic illnesses or the death of partners or friends. Here in Florida, we sometimes refer to it as "God's waiting room" given the percentage of older people who migrate here to retire. The death of a spouse or diagnosis of a serious illness motivates many of my patients to seek therapy. They can no longer avoid confronting their own mortality and that of those they love.

With many patients, talking about death is an unavoidable topic; it's inevitably lurking in the background when we're desperate, grieving, or depressed. When talking about death and dying, I caution students and interns to avoid platitudes and vague terms about death like "passing" or religious terms like "going to heaven." It's a struggle to bring up an issue that we know is painful to talk about, that brings up so many strong feelings, difficult memories, and anxious foreboding for both our patients and us. To ignore the topic when a patient is grieving or seriously ill communicates that we are uncomfortable and avoidant. If we are anxious about death, our patients will protect us by not bringing up the issue. Our own existential anxiety can't get in the way if we are to help others confront the issue of dying.

Yalom (2017) notes that "…learning to live well is to learn to die well." (p. 125). I agree with his recommendation that we approach anxious patients by inviting them to have a matter-of-fact dialogue about the nature of their anxiety and the specific concerns they have about death. Do they fear becoming dependent? Were they close to someone who had a particularly painful death? Are they concerned about someone they will leave behind? I have usually found it to be the case that "there is a correlation between the degree of death anxiety and the degree one has fulfilled oneself" (Yalom, 2017, p. 15). The patient who is on the "despair" side of Erik Erikson's (1980) final stage of development offers us an opportunity to help them become more actualized, more of who they want to be, even at the end. Integrity at this stage of life is characterized by composure, broadmindedness, appropriate emotional forbearance, and peace of mind. Encouraging patients to examine and confront their fears and regrets is how we walk together on the path to greater peace of mind as we approach death.

Suicide

The death of a patient through suicide is particularly challenging for therapists. It is one of the most painful experiences we face in the big chair. "Approximately 50 percent of senior therapists have faced suicide, or a serious suicide attempt, of a current or past patient." (Yalom, 2017 p. 253). Those of us who have been in the big chair for several decades have most likely faced the threat or completion of suicide several times over. It's an experience that comes with the territory, particularly with vulnerable populations like drug abusers and addicts, those with severe depression, psychosis, or eating disorders, and people who have sunken into despair. We work with high-risk populations for suicide. It's imperative that psychotherapists and counselors have appropriate and repeated training in intervening with patients who are suicidal and that we have resources for support and assistance when we lose a patient.

My first job in the field in 1973 was at a state hospital in Austin, Texas on a unit for severely mentally ill patients. Several months after I began working there, we admitted a woman in her mid-20s who was profoundly depressed and suicidal. Jane was admitted involuntarily and began using any means she could to try and harm herself including attempting to stab herself with a butter knife and running down hallways and slamming into walls. In order to prevent her from harm, she was placed in an observation room, an actual padded cell with no furniture, just a mattress on the floor without sheets because we feared she would try to strangle herself. When she ate, she was given plastic silverware and two attendants stayed in the room with her until she finished. We observed her every 20 minutes to make sure that she was okay. She seemed to calm down after several hours and an injection of tranquilizers. Staff entered the seclusion room to take her to the toilet or bring her food and, after about 8 hours, she was cooperative and engaged in more conversation than she had since she was admitted to the hospital. When asked about her suicidal intentions, she simply stated that she was feeling better. After about 15 hours in the observation room, she asked one of the staff if she could have her journal and a pencil. Her request was granted and when she was next observed 20 minutes later, Jane was dead. She was my first encounter with death by suicide.

Suicide Assessment

Knowing how do to a suicide risk assessment is as important for all mental health professionals as knowing how to take blood pressure and temperature are for medical professionals. At present, I teach classes for freshmen and sophomore students in Human Services. In several of my classes, we focus on doing a basic suicide assessment so that they know how to interact more effectively with people who are potentially suicidal. I also made it a requirement for students to complete the Adult and Youth Mental Health First Aid USA courses, trainings developed to prepare both professionals and members of the public to effectively assess and intervene in mental health emergencies including the threat of suicide (Mental Health Association of Maryland, Inc., 2012, www.MentalHealthFirstAid.org) . These trainings are offered throughout the United States, often through local chapters of the National Alliance on Mental Illness (NAMI). I encourage everyone to take the course. The goal of these courses is to emulate what was done with CPR (cardiopulmonary resuscitation) trainings and educate as many people as possible to learn to interact humanely and effectively with someone in a psychiatric emergency. No one who occupies the big chair can be unaware of or misinformed about how to assess and intervene with a suicidal patient.

When assessing suicide risk, we must be precise in our language. That point was brought home when I was supervising a graduate student at the counseling center at the University of Colorado at Denver. We operated a community clinic with our students who received live supervision from faculty through a one-way mirror via a phone connected to the observation room behind the mirror. I was observing the session through the mirror with several students from our counseling techniques class. A student trainee was conducting an intake interview with a new patient to the clinic, a woman in her mid-forties who had been referred by a friend who was concerned about symptoms of depression. As the student was going through the protocol for an intake and gathering needed information, it seemed she was avoiding asking the patient about suicidal ideation or intent despite the woman affirming that she had been feeling deeply depressed for several months. I phoned in to the student that she needed to do a suicide assessment to determine if this patient might be at risk. All our students had learned the suicide assessment protocol in class prior to approving students to work in the clinic. I requested she "Please ask the patient if she is thinking about suicide and if so, determine the level of risk." The student looked anxious after I gave her the instruction, but turned to the patient and asked, "Are you thinking about doing something to yourself?" The woman looked confused for a moment then looked at the student and said, "Do you mean like masturbating?" Be precise! You can't sneak up on the question of suicidal risk.

So long as a patient remains engaged in the session, I seek to find a way to work together and get past the threat of suicide. An assessment is vital in determining the level of urgency and to help plan what to do to avoid a suicide attempt. I think of assessing suicidal intent as similar to assessing whether or not someone is going on vacation. If someone admits to thinking about suicide, the first step is determining whether there's a plan. The more detailed the plan, the more likely they are to carry it out. If the patient has a clear plan of when, where, and how, has the means to carry out that plan, and is determined to do so or they are so impaired that they can't commit to a no-suicide agreement, then the level is extremely high that they will make an attempt. Patients who say, "I just want to say goodbye to you" or "It's no use trying to talk me out of this" are waving warning flags and, at that point, my commitment is to intervene to protect them if they can't commit to alternatives to a suicide attempt.

A serious threat of suicide means that I can break confidentiality and place the patient under an involuntary commitment or, especially in the case of minors, alert family members and determine if there are supportive relatives who are willing and able to do a 24 hour watch to prevent a suicide attempt. I've had to intervene in those ways on a few occasions, always with great reluctance but with a clear focus on trying to save someone's life. If possible, I keep the patient engaged in that process and explain exactly what I intend to do and what they can expect to happen. I'll stay with a patient until they are with other professionals or family who can provide a safe environment for them. It's always a very challenging situation for both the patient and me and often compromises the therapeutic relationship we have. I'm certainly willing to trade that for helping someone survive a suicidal crisis.

Stay Connected

So long as there is not an imminent threat of suicide, I work to stay connected to the patient. As Cozolino (2004) reminds us, "...strategy Number One: Don't panic!" (p. 42). I can't be helpful to someone else in crisis if I'm overwhelmed by fear or anxiety. That's true any time we're interacting with someone who is especially challenging: They're reporting abuse or trauma, exhibiting psychotic symptoms such as delusions or hallucinations, threatening to harm you or others, expressing sexual interest in you, or engaged in particularly risky behaviors (e.g., driving while intoxicated, self-mutilation). I find suicide is often the most anxiety provoking because it feels like such an enormous challenge from the patient to say or do something that will convince them to stay alive. I must connect deeply to my own beliefs and values: That life is worth living, that crises will pass, feelings will change, and despair can be relieved over time. I'm on the side of life, without equivocation.

It's important to understand that only a small minority of people who are considering suicide go on to make an attempt. I work with the ambivalence. Deciding to kill oneself is not easy for most people, any more than it would be to decide to kill someone else. The best example of that ambivalence was an experience I had on a suicide prevention hotline, a service we provided through the community mental health center where I worked in west Texas. I trained and supervised volunteers who answered the hot line calls. One evening, we received a call from a man who was a frequent caller, usually when he was intoxicated. He was also a patient at the center, so we had information about him including where he lived and that he was being treated for depression and alcoholism. On this particular evening, his voice was slurred and instead of engaging in his usual rambling conversation with the volunteer, he said "I just wanted to call and thank ya'll for all the time you spent listening to me. Tonight's the end for me, I can't do this anymore. I just wanted to say thanks and goodbye." I asked the volunteer to try and keep him on the line while I went to call the sheriff to go to the man's apartment and do a wellness check. I informed the dispatcher that we knew the man had loaded guns at his apartment and that he sounded very intoxicated. Our caller had hung up on the volunteer after sharing with her that he did have his gun all ready and was just going to finish his bottle of Jack Daniel's and end his pain.

When we tried to call back, he wouldn't pick up the phone. After about 45 minutes, we got a call from the sheriff who was laughing and said, "You're not going to believe this one." He had taken a rookie officer with him to the man's apartment: Both were aware that this was a high-risk situation with an intoxicated man who was probably holding a loaded gun. He wanted the rookie to take the lead, so when they were at the man's door, the rookie shouted, "Police officers, we're coming in," kicked open the door and ran in. Our caller was on the couch in the front room, a pistol in one hand and a bottle of whiskey in the other. The rookie officer pulled out his gun and yelled, "Stop or I'll shoot." The suicidal man calmly put down the gun and bottle, put his hands in the air, stood up and went with the officers to their car and to the psychiatric hospital for evaluation and treatment. That's the power of ambivalence.

I pay close attention to the moment we're in if a patient says they are considering suicide. If a person is fully intent on committing suicide, then why are they sitting and talking with me instead of out making an attempt? I share that question with suicidal patients and ask, "What helped you decide to take the time to talk with me about your suicidal feelings instead of being somewhere else trying to kill yourself?" I want to know what is making the decision difficult for them and use that information to help me tip the ambivalence toward staying alive. Until someone makes an attempt, your best ally is the struggle between life and death that is going on in the person. If they have children or other family members or friends that would be deeply hurt by losing them to suicide, I want to make those concerns foremost in their minds. I've worked with the children of people who committed suicide and I share with suicidal patients the despair that often persists in the lives of those children and the increased likelihood that they will consider suicide when encountering problems in their lives. If religious beliefs that prohibit suicide are part of their values, I emphasize the importance of trusting the tenets of their faith.

I sometimes share stories of people who survived their suicide attempts and were grateful to be alive such as Robert whose story is at the end of the chapter. I might also talk about people who were seriously injured or disabled because of their attempts. I worked on a neuro-rehab unit during my doctoral internship so have some pretty graphic examples including several patients who shot themselves in the head, a man who stabbed himself in the heart, and a woman who jumped from a high bridge and survived. I make it clear that those individuals survived but were never going to be the same. Only one in twenty-five people who make a suicide attempt will die from that attempt (Suicide Awareness Voices of Education, 2020). I also share that information to challenge the fantasy that all attempts lead to death. Most don't. I want to do whatever I can do to add weight to the "staying alive" part of the ambivalence and make the "killing myself" part less attractive.

It's also important to appreciate that the vast majority of people who entertain the thought of suicide don't want to die, they're looking for relief from what feels like an unbearable time in their life. The good news about suicide intervention is that the odds are strongly in our favor of being able to help people get past that deep despair and instead work toward having a better life. Working with suicidal people is risky, but like many risky endeavors, the rewards are great when we are able to accompany someone as they move through that desperate time and find the light on the other side of the darkness. Surviving and even thriving after a period of suicidal crisis can build resilience and determination to change ourselves in ways that help us not to fall into the pit of despair that makes us question our willingness to exist. Making a choice to stay alive can be linked to a choice to work toward a life we live more fully. That's what I strive to help patients learn, that what seemed to be the end can become a new beginning.

The Hardest Letting Go

It's almost inevitable that at some point in our professional lives, we will lose a patient to suicide. When I've had talks with colleagues about patients who have ended their lives, it's always the case that those are the ghosts that haunt us most. Questions about "What did I miss?" or "What else could I have done?" stay with me when I remember those I lost to suicidal despair. Talking to colleagues and finding a therapist for myself have been so helpful during those times. That's probably what kept me in the profession when I felt like such a failure and had difficulty trusting my judgment and abilities. A patient committing suicide is what we fear most and with good reason. Deaths of patients from overdose, homicide, or other incidents are usually accidental or unintended: Not so with suicide. I feel what friends and family feel when a patient dies from suicide – helpless, angry, ashamed, and guilty. Also, there's an overwhelming, desperate sadness, and an obsession with what I did or didn't do that led to the death of a patient. It's a lesson in letting go that is very hard to accept.

I can't imagine going through that experience without support and consultation with colleagues, many of whom have also lost patients along the way. Also, the therapists who let me grieve and rant and do what we do to heal from loss were extraordinarily helpful in saying goodbye to the 23-year-old mother of two who suffered from severe bi-polar disorder and drowned herself in the family swimming pool, the 14-year-old boy who had been bullied past the point of his endurance and shot himself with his father's gun, and the 56-year-old man who relapsed after 12 years of sobriety and overdosed rather than face another round of addiction. I appreciate all the help I had in letting go of those souls and finding renewed hope in all the other patients who made it through to the other side. They helped teach me the courage to go on and continue to help others. I'm deeply grateful to everyone who renewed my hope.

NOTES FROM THE BIG CHAIR

It's rare to meet a senior therapist who has not lost patients to one or more of these circumstances: Domestic violence, eating disorders, overdose, murder, or suicide. We also lose patients through accidents or natural causes, both unexpected and anticipated deaths. Psychotherapists regularly confront death or the threat of death in their work. There is no place to hide if you occupy the big chair; you will be required to face your own mortality and that of others. Death, simply put, is the end of hope, the impossibility of further possibility. When there is no way to avoid their pain, I hope that my patient and I can find a way to bring greater compassion, wisdom, and acceptance to their suffering. I feel honored to bear witness and lend support to the resilience and determination of so many people. Being present with other's pain has certainly helped me become more respectful of the overwhelming circumstances that people face. I appreciate the courage and grace of those who get up every day and do what they can to take care of themselves and others. I hope to be one of those people for many years to come.

Lessons from the Big Chair: Chapter 10

- Facing death is the final lesson in letting go; letting go of everything that we have and that we are.
- Psychotherapists work with high-risk populations and must learn to make peace with dying if we are to help others face death.
- The hardest aspect of being a psychotherapist is losing a patient.
- The top concerns when death is imminent are the dying process or conditions, being pain free, and emotional well-being.
- It's imperative that all therapists be trained in conducting a suicide risk assessment and in techniques to intervene and prevent a suicide attempt.

- We are good at preventing suicide. Most people who share with a therapist that they are suicidal will not go on to make an attempt.
- At some point, you will lose a patient to suicide. When you do, get help and talk with your colleagues.

Case Study: Robert

Robert was a 24-year-old man whom I was seeing at a community mental health clinic in a small town in west Texas. I had recently graduated with my master's degree in counseling psychology and had been with the center for almost two years. I was the director of the crisis intervention/suicide prevention hotline and saw patients on an outpatient basis. Robert had called the crisis line a few days before my first meeting with him. When I met Robert for the intake, I was impressed with his intelligence and gentle demeanor. His sadness filled the room and I was aware of how difficult the interview was for him as he struggled to share what had happened.

Robert was engaged to be married to Sharon who he had been with for all his adult life. They met during their freshman year at the university in our town. She was the first and only love of his life. He had not had any girlfriends in high school because he was very focused on academics and had plans to become an attorney. Robert came from a middle-class family that settled in our small Texas town several generations before. His parents had been high school sweethearts, happily married for over 30 years. Robert was their only child and was much beloved by his family. He spent most of his time at his fiancé's apartment since their engagement two years previous.

Approximately three weeks before his call to our hotline, without any warning, Sharon called off their wedding. Despite his pleas, she offered no reason for her decision and was unwilling to talk with him about trying to reconcile. She refused all contact with Robert after her confrontation, she changed her phone number and the lock on her apartment. Clothing and other belongings of his that were at her place were returned to his parents' home by an anonymous person. Sharon was gone.

Robert moved back into his room at his parent's house. It was his last year at the university and he tried to continue going to classes but couldn't concentrate and did very poorly on an important exam. He would sometimes see his former fiancé on campus, always in the company of friends. The one time that he tried to approach Sharon, she angrily told him to stay away and one of the friends with her threatened to call campus security if he bothered her again.

As Robert shared information with me, he struggled to speak through his tears. Nothing in his life had prepared him for the pain he experienced from this unexpected loss. He had stopped going to classes, isolated himself in his room at home, and refused to see friends because he felt so ashamed and confused. Repeatedly, he asked "Why did she do this?" When I asked what he meant by "do this" he said, "She erased my future."

He was the embodiment of someone who felt hopeless and helpless, two red flags for suicide. In assessing his suicide potential, he admitted to other warning signs: He withdrew from contact with family and friends, he couldn't eat or sleep, he began bingeing on alcohol to numb his pain, and he felt certain that he would never feel happy again. His family physician prescribed Valium to reduce his anxiety and help him sleep. I was also aware that there had recently been a completed suicide by another student at the university. When I asked Robert about it, he didn't know the young man, but had heard the rumor that it was because of a relationship breakup. Most importantly, when I asked about suicidal ideation, he admitted having thoughts about ending his life but didn't have a plan. Robert agreed to a no suicide contract for his safety and we met several more times over two weeks. He was able to resume going to classes but remained very isolated and depressed.

On week three, Robert missed his appointment with me. Instead of seeing him at the office, I received a call from his distraught mother that Robert was in critical care at our local hospital after overdosing on Valium and alcohol the previous night. They had found him early that morning, unconscious, with the empty liquor and Valium bottles on his nightstand. I went to see him at the hospital. He was unconscious, surrounded by wires, tubes, and beeping machines. The staff who were caring for him were uncertain if he would survive. I was devastated. Although I had worked with other patients who were suicidal, I hadn't yet lost anyone that I had worked with in therapy. I said my goodbyes to Robert and was filled with regret that I hadn't been able to help him through this crisis. After forty years in the field, I still remember the horrible feeling that I missed something that could have prevented his attempt.

As I was getting ready to leave, a young woman came in to see Robert. When she asked who I was, I said I was a friend of Roberts. She was a friend of both Robert and Sharon. She was visibly upset and said she had been with Robert the previous evening and felt responsible for what had happened. He ran into her after a late afternoon class and pleaded with her to talk to him about what happened with Sharon. She shared with him that Sharon had fallen in love with another man she met in one of her classes and that they had already moved in together. She had been involved with the new boyfriend for several months before she ended the relationship with Robert.

This was a blow that Robert didn't know how to absorb. He went home, started drinking and, at some point late that night, swallowed a nearly full bottle of Valium. Despite our agreement, he didn't try to call the hotline or let his parents know he was suicidal. Not only had he lost his future, his past was destroyed as well. The deception was the final insult; it was simply too much for him.

I was also overwhelmed. I didn't go back to see Robert again, nor did I contact his parents. I couldn't bring myself to risk hearing he had died. This was a new experience for me as well. I had never gone through a significant loss, either personally or professionally. My supervisor was very supportive and compassionate. We reviewed the case and completed a report for his file. The supervisor took over my responsibilities as the hotline director and reduced my caseload. I avoided taking cases where there was a good possibility of suicidal ideation or behavior. I didn't know if Robert would recover. I didn't know if I would either. I started therapy for myself and found it essential for staying in the field. I stayed alive as a therapist and switched to working in a different program at the mental health center.

Three years later, I was in my office at the center and the receptionist called to say there was a gentleman asking for me at the desk. I had her send him back. It was Robert. In his arms was a baby girl only a few months old. I began crying and apologizing; I told him I didn't know if he had survived and was so grateful to see that he was alive. He introduced me to his daughter. He said that when he awoke in the hospital, his first thought was how much he regretted his suicide attempt. The hospital provided a therapist with whom he worked for many months and who helped him come to terms with what had happened with Sharon. He finished his degree and began dating a woman he met at his first job. They fell in love, married, and started a family. Robert came to see me to let me know he was sorry for the suicide attempt and regretted not talking with me about what had happened. I apologized too for not being able to help him enough to prevent his suicide attempt. We hugged and wished each other well. To this day, I am so grateful to Robert for coming to see me and let me know that his story hadn't ended. In fact, Robert was happy. So was I.

Lesson from the Big Chair: Hope

I wanted to end this chapter with a story of hope. My experience with Robert has been enormously valuable in helping me through the loss of other patients over the years. I'm so grateful for his thoughtfulness in coming to see me that day, it was such a profoundly moving and unusual experience. I rarely know where the story goes after a patient who is suicidal leaves therapy. Having an experience like I did with Robert reminds me of the importance and resilience of hope. When I know a patient is at risk and I lose my connection with them, I can think of Robert and be hopeful that there is a chapter in their story that changes the patient for the better.

AFTERWORD

I began writing this book in May 2019 and am writing this final piece in May 2020. A change unlike any in my lifetime began in January 2020 when the world started to feel the impact of the COVID-19 pandemic. At several points in the book, I have gone back and inserted some information about how this global challenge may be likely to impact the profession of psychotherapy, those of us who are practitioners, and most importantly, the patients that we serve. I trust that by the time this book is published, much more will have changed.

I've long been a student of chaos and complexity theory in physics and how some of those concepts apply to our particular science of psychology and the work that we do as psychotherapists. More than two decades ago, my colleagues Dr. Michael Butz and Dr. William McCown and I explored those ideas and wrote about the disruptive nature of chaos and crisis as a source of change and reorganization (Butz, Chamberlain, & McCown, 1997; Chamberlain & Butz, 1998). One of the tenets of chaos theory concerns sensitive dependence on initial conditions, often referred to as the "Butterfly Effect," which describes the transformative potential of even a small disruption in an interactive system like the weather or human relationships. "Open systems not only can move from chaos to an adaptive new order but can be unstable enough for a small variable to completely change their behavior over time" (Butz, Chamberlain & McCown, 1997, p. 62). Another part of complexity theory describes the irreversibility of how dynamic, interactive systems function. I like to think of it as the idea that you can't unscramble eggs. Events or processes that change us or our circumstances change the course of our experience and environment. You don't get to go back to start. I strongly believe that we are in the midst of creating a "new normal" in our profession in the coming years.

A month ago, I transitioned my practice to my home and began doing sessions by phone as I looked into options for telehealth video formats. The college where I teach closed our classrooms in spring mid-semester and we're not planning to open until after the first of the year, if then. My only human contact not mediated by a phone or computer screen or a face mask at a distance of at least six feet is with my partner, Jeff, for whom I am so grateful. I'm struggling with how to be a psychotherapist and to train others who are coming into this profession without being in person with them. The flow of conversation and the ability to observe all the nonverbal behavior that is so informative is altered in a way that I'm not sure how to process. I greatly miss how being in a therapy office or a classroom provides a much bigger setting to observe and interact than a screen allows. In some ways, I feel as if I'm relearning how to do psychotherapy.

I'm hopeful that this period of chaos will transform both our profession and our culture. I'm looking forward to being a student again as I learn how to best serve patients and students with whom I can't be in direct contact. In the longer term, I am curious to see if this becomes an opportunity for substantive, systematic change. Can we bring the importance of mental health care to the forefront? In the coming months, we will be called upon to meet the needs of our medical colleagues who are undergoing enormous trauma in treating so many patients who die. We will be faced with patients who are deeply impacted by loss and grief, who are faced with the need to rebuild their lives, and who find that anxiety, depression, and other mental and emotional challenges they may have been experiencing are magnified through this crisis. Those of us in the big chairs will have much important work to do.

I have so many questions and am longing for conversations with colleagues and students about where this change can take us. I think it's time to begin a new book, one that examines how we might be able to emerge from this chaos with a new paradigm for our work. I wish all my readers safe passage through this difficult time, and please share your thoughts with me on my bigchair.blog.

All the best – Linda Chamberlain

REFERENCES

Aiken, G. A. (2006). *The potential effect of mindfulness meditation on the cultivation of empathy in psychotherapy*. Ph.D. thesis, Saybrook Graduate School and Research Center, San Francisco, CA.

Alcoholics Anonymous. (2001). *Alcoholics Anonymous, 4th Edition*. New York: A.A. World Services.

American Psychiatric Association (2013). *Diagnostic and Statistical Manual of Mental Disorders*, (5th ed.). Arlington, VA: American Psychiatric Association.

American Psychological Association (May 3, 2005). The role of psychologists in end-or-life decisions and quality of care. Retrieved from https://www.apa.org/research/action/end.

Anderson, H.C. (1844). *New Fairy Tales*. Copenhagen, Denmark: C.A. Reitzel.

Baum, L. F. (1900). *The Wonderful Wizard of Oz*. New York: Sweetwater Press.

Becker, E. (1973). *The Denial of Death*. Blencoe, IL: Free Press.

Bike, D. H., Horcross, J. C., & Schatz, D. M. (2009). Processes and outcomes of psychotherapists' personal therapy: Replication and extension 20 years later. *Psychotherapy: Theory, Research, Practice, Training*, 46(1), 19–31.

Bishop, S., Lau, M., Shapiro, S., Carlson, L., Anderson, N., & Carmody, J. (2004). Mindfulness: A proposed operational definition. *Clinical Psychology: Science and Practice*, 11, 230–241.

Bozarth, J. D. (2013). Unconditional positive regard. In M. Cooper, M. O'Hara, P. F. Schmid, & A. C. Bohart (Eds.), *The Handbook of Person-Centred Psychotherapy and Counselling* (pp. 180–192). New York: Palgrave Macmillan. Retrieved from http://dx.doi.org/10.1007/978-1-137-32900-4_12.

Bugaeff, P. B. (2018). *Tell Me About It: Memoir of A Psychotherapist.* Ant Press: Retrieved from www.antpress.org.

Burgess, A. (1962). *A Clockwork Orange.* New York: Norton Critical Edition.

Butz, M. R., Chamberlain, L. L., & McCown, W. G. (1997). *Strange Attractors: Chaos, Complexity, and the Art of Family Therapy.* New York: Wiley.

Chamberlain, L. & Butz, M. (1998). *Clinical Chaos: A Therapist's Guide to Nonlinear Dynamics and Therapeutic Change.* Philadelphia, PA: Brunner/Mazel.

Claxton, G. (1999). *The Heart of Buddhism: Practical Wisdom for an Agitated World.* London: Thorsons.

Keyes C. L. M., Eisenberg D., Perry G. S., Dube S. R. , Kroenke K., & Dhingra S. S. (2012) The relationship of level of positive mental health with current mental disorders in predicting suicidal behavior and academic impairment in college students. *Journal of American College Health,* 60(2), 126–133, doi: 10.1080/07448481.2011.608393

Cozolino, L. (2004). *The Making of a Therapist: A Practical Guide for the Inner Journey.* New York: W.W. Norton.

Lama D. (2004). *Many Ways to Nirvana.* New York: Penguin Compass.

Delle, S. (February, 2017). There's no shame in taking care of your mental health. Ted Talks. Retrieved from https://www.ted.com/talks/sangu_delle_there_s_no_shame_in_taking_care_of_your_mental_health?language=en.

Dixon, M. R., Nastally, B. L., & Waterman, A. (2010). The effect of gambling activities on happiness levels of nursing home residents. *Journal of Applied Behaviour Analysis. 43,* 531–535.

Duncan, B. L. (2014). *On Becoming a Better Therapist* (2nd Ed.). Washington, DC: American Psychological Organization.

Duncan, B. L., Miller, S. D., Wampold, B. E., & Hubble, M. A. (2010). *The Heart and Soul of Change: Delivering What Works in Psychotherapy* (2nd Ed.). Washington, DC: American Psychological Association.

Erikson, E. (1980). *Identity and the Life Cycle.* New York: W.W. Norton & Company.

Farrell, L. (March, 2018). Understanding the relationship between subjective wellbeing and gambling behavior. *Journal of Gambling Studies,* 34:1, 55–71.

Frankl, V. E. (1959). *Man's Search for Meaning.* Boston: Beacon Press.

Ghent, E. (1999). Masochism, submission, surrender: Masochism as a perversion of surrender. In S. Mitchell &L. Aron (Eds.) *Relational Psychoanalysis: The Emergence of Tradition* (pp.211–242). Hillsdale, NJ: Analytic Press.

Gilbert, M. (2019). The role of trauma in addiction. *Vineland National Center.* Retrieved October 2, 2019 from http://www.vinlandcenter.org/trauma-addiction/

Goldberg, A. (2012). *An Analysis of Failure: An Investigation of Failed Cases in Psychoanalysis and Psychotherapy.* New York: Routledge.

Gottlieb, L. (2019). *Maybe You Should Talk to Someone.* Boston: Harper Houghton Mifflin Company.

Hari, J. (June, 2015). Everything you think you know about addiction is wrong. *Ted Talks.* Retrieved from https://www.ted.com/talks/johann_hari_everything_you_think_you_know_about_addiction_is_wrong.

Heylighen F. (1992). Principles of systems and cybernetics: An evolutionary perspective. In Trappl, R. (Ed.) *Cybernetics and Systems 92* (pp.3–10). Singapore: World Science.

Hick, S. F. & Bien, T. (Eds.) (2008). *Mindfulness and the Therapeutic Relationship.* New York: The Guilford Press.

Hoglend, P. A., Monsen, J. T., & Ronnestad, M. H. (2013). The contribution of the quality of therapists' personal lives to the development of the working alliance. *Journal of Counseling Psychology, 60*(4), 483–495.

Hunt, M., Marx, R., Lipson, C., & Young, J. (2018). No more FOMO: Limiting social media decreases loneliness and depression. *Journal of Social and Clinical Psychology, 37*(10), 751–768. Retrieved from https://doi.org/10.1521/jscp.2018.37.10.751.

Kabat-Zinn, J. (1994). *Wherever You Go There You Are: Mindfulness Meditation in Everyday Life.* New York: Hyperion.

Kornfield, J. (2008). *The Wise Heart: A Guide to the Universal Teachings of Buddhist Psychology.* New York: Bantam Books.

Kottler, J. (2017). *On Being a Therapist,* (5th ed.) New York: Oxford University Press.

Kottler, J. & Carlson, J. (2014). *On being a master therapist: Practicing what you preach.* Hoboken, New Jersey: John Wiley & Sons.

Lander, L. (2004). *The Lost Art of Compassion.* San Francisco: Zondervan.

Lakhiani, V. (YouTube) (Feb. 13, 2013). The 6 phase guided meditation. Retrieved from https://youtu.be/EaRu14P9H84 .

Linehan, M. (2020). *Building a Life Worth Living: A Memoir.* New York: Random House.

Mathieu, F. (2012). *The Compassion Fatigue Workbook.* New York: Routledge.

Martin, D. G. (2016). *Counseling & Therapy Skills* (4th ed.). Long Grove, IL: Waveland Press, Inc.

McCown, W. & Chamberlain, L. (2000). *Best Possible Odds: Contemporary Treatment Strategies for Gambling Disorders.* New York: John Wiley & Sons, Inc.

Meier, E. A., Gallegos, J. V., Thomas, L. P., Depp, C. A., Irwin, S. A., & Jeste, D. V. (2016). Defining a Good Death (Successful Dying): Literature Review and a Call for Research and Public Dialogue. *The American Journal of Geriatric Psychiatry,* 24(4), 261–271. doi:10.1016/j.jagp.2016.01.135.

Mental Health Association of Maryland, Inc. (2012). *Mental Health First Aid USA.* Lutherville, MD: Mental Health Association of Maryland, Inc. Retrieved from www.MentalHealthFirstAid.org.

MentalHealth.gov (2017). Mental health myths and facts. Retrieved from https://www.mentalhealth.gov/basics/mental-health-myths-facts

Miller, W.R. & Rollnick S. (1991). *Motivational Interviewing: Preparing People to Change Addictive Behavior.* New York: Guilford Press.

Mongrain, M., Chin, J.M., & Shapira, L.B. (2011). Practicing Compassion Increases Happiness and Self-Esteem. *Journal of Happiness Studies,* 12, 963–981, doi:10.1007/s10902-010-9239-1.

National Opinion Research Center, General Social Survey (2014). University of Chicago, Chicago, IL, USA.

Nissen-Lie, H. A., Havik, O. E., Hoglend, P. A., Monsen, J. T., & Ronnestad, M. H. (2013). The contribution of the quality of therapists 'personal lives to the development of a working alliance. *Journal of Counseling Psychology,* 60(4), 483–495.

Pilgrim, D., Rogers, A., & Bentall, R. (2009). The centrality of personal relationships in the creation and amelioration of mental health problems: the current interdisciplinary case. *Health,* 13, 235–254. Retrieved October 22, 2009, from https://journals.sagepub.com/doi/abs/10.1177/1363459308099686.

Pipher, M. (2016). *Letters to a Young Therapist.* New York: Basic Books.

Prochaska, J.O., DiClemente, C.C., & Norcross, J.C. (1992). In search of how people change: Applications to the addictive behaviors. *American Psychologist, 47,* 1102–1114.

Rogers, C. (1961). *On Becoming a Person.* Boston: Houghton Mifflin Company.

Rubin, G. (2009), *The Happiness Project.* New York: Harper Collins.

Saks, E. (June, 2012). A tale of mental illness – from the inside. *Ted Talks.* Retrieved from https://www.ted.com/talks/elyn_saks_a_tale_of_mental_illness_from_the_inside.

Seligman, M. E. P. (2002). *Authentic Happiness: Using the New Positive Psychology to Realize Your Potential for Lasting Fulfillment.* New York: Free Press.

Seppala, E., (2016). *The Happiness Track: How to Apply the Science of Happiness to Accelerate Your Success.* New York: Harper Collins Publishers.

Shapiro, F. (2018). *Eye Movement Desensitization and Reprocessing (EMDR) Therapy,* 3rd Ed. New York: Guilford Press.

Suicide Awareness Voices of Education: SAVE (2020). Retrieved from https://save.org/about-suicide/suicide-facts/

Tartakovsky, M. (2019). Media's Damaging Depictions of Mental Illness. *Psych Central.* Retrieved on October 18, 2019, from https://psychcentral.com/lib/medias-damaging-depictions-of-mental-illness/

Three approaches to psychotherapy. All three session (1965). Retrieved from https://youtu.be/5errJ-u2_eg

Vonnegut, K. (1987). *Bluebeard.* New York: Dell Publishing.

W., Bill. (1976). *Alcoholics Anonymous: The Story of How Many Thousands of Men and Women Have Recovered from Alcoholism.* New York: Alcoholics Anonymous World Services.

Watkins, P. C., McLaughlin, T., & Parker, J. P. (2019). Gratitude and subjective well-being: Cultivating gratitude for a harvest of happiness. In N. Silton (Ed.), *Scientific Concepts Behind Happiness, Kindness, and Empathy in Contemporary Society* (pp. 20–42). Hershey, PA: IGI Global. doi:10.4018/978-1-5225-5918-4.ch002

Westra, H. (n.d.). The effectiveness of psychotherapy: What the research tells us. *National Register of Health Service Psychologists.* Retrieved from https://www.findapsychologist.org/the-effectiveness-of-psychotherapy-what-the-research-tells-us-by-dr-henry-westra/

Wheat, P. (2005, January). *Mindfulness meditation: Promoting cultural competency. Spectrum*, pp. 18–19. Retrieved from www.spectrumjournal.ca/index.php/spectrum

Wilber, K. (1981). *No Boundary*. London: Shambhala.

Yalom, I. (2002). *The gift of therapy: An open letter to a new generation of therapists and their patients*. New York: Harper

Yalom, I (2017). *Becoming myself: A psychiatrist's memoir*. New York: Basic Books.

ABOUT THE AUTHOR

Linda Chamberlain is a Licensed Psychologist and Professor of Human Services at Pasco-Hernando State College in New Port Richey, Florida. Linda also served on the faculty at the University of Denver, University of Colorado at Denver, Regis University and the University of South Florida. She has worked as a psychotherapist, educator, trainer, and supervisor for more than 40 years. Linda has been a clinician in both public and private hospitals and clinics and maintains a private practice with specialties in addiction recovery, gambling disorders, relationship counseling, trauma recovery, and treatment of anxiety and depression.

She is also a member and clinical consultant with Bikers Against Child Abuse (BACA), Bay Bridges Chapter in Florida.

Dr. Chamberlain has coauthored and contributed to several books on chaos theory including *Strange Attractors: Chaos, Complexity, and the Art of Family Therapy*, *Clinical Chaos: A Therapist's Guide to Nonlinear Dynamics and Therapeutic Change*, and *Chaos theory in Psychology and the Life Sciences*. She is coauthor with Dr. William McCown of a book on problem gambling, *Best Possible Odds: Contemporary Treatment Strategies for Gambling Disorders*, and contributed chapters to the *Handbook of Addictive Disorders: A Practical Guide to Diagnosis and Treatment, Substance Abuse Counseling: Theory and Practice,* and the *Handbook of Couple and Family Assessment.* Linda has been a speaker and trainer at numerous conferences in the United States, Canada, Japan, and Holland. In 2019, she created bigchair.blog as a resource for connection and digital conversation with other therapists.

INDEX

For Product Safety Concerns and Information please contact our EU
representative GPSR@taylorandfrancis.com
Taylor & Francis Verlag GmbH, Kaufingerstraße 24, 80331 München, Germany